NO-FUSS DIABETIC COOKBOOK FOR BEGINNERS

Taste Meets Health with Endless Mouthwatering, Low-Carb & Low-Glycemic Meals to Help Manage Diabetes and Prediabetes with Ease | 49-Day Meal Plan Included

Elodie Vance

TABLE OF CONTENTS

OPENING THOUGHTS 9

   Embracing Change Post-50 9

   Understanding Diabetes in Your Golden Years 11

   The Power of Diet in Diabetes Management 12

   Setting Realistic Goals 14

NAVIGATING THE DIABETIC DIET LANDSCAPE 16

   Deciphering Nutritional Needs After 50 16

   The Do's and Don'ts: Foods for Diabetes 18

   Balancing Blood Sugar with Smart Eating 19

   Unearthing Hidden Sugars in Everyday Foods 21

WELLNESS AND WHOLESOME INGREDIENTS 23

   Superfoods for Diabetic Health 23

   Sourcing and Selecting Quality Ingredients 25

   The Role of Organic and Non-GMO Foods 26

   Understanding Food Labels and Claims 28

REVITALIZING BREAKFAST RECIPES 30

     Savory Mushroom and Spinach Frittata 31

     Almond and Coconut Chia Pudding 31

     Zesty Tomato and Avocado Toast 32

     Herbed Turkey and Spinach Mini Quiches 32

     Chia and Coconut Yogurt Parfait 33

     Savory Spinach and Mushroom Egg Muffins 33

     Cinnamon Almond Flax Pancakes 34

     Zucchini and Herb Breakfast Hash 34

     Zucchini and Bell Pepper Mini Frittatas 35

     Chia and Berry Yogurt Parfait 35

     Spinach and Feta Breakfast Wrap 36

     Almond Butter and Banana Open Sandwich 36

     Savory Cottage Cheese Bowl 37

     Almond Flour Pancakes with Berry Compote 37

     Savory Spinach and Feta Muffins 38

     Smoked Salmon and Avocado Wrap 38

     Spinach and Feta Breakfast Wraps 39

     Almond Butter and Banana Toast 39

     Zucchini and Goat Cheese Frittata 40

     Almond Flour Blueberry Pancakes 40

     Shakshuka with Spinach and Feta 41

     Coconut Yogurt Parfait with Kiwi and Walnuts 41

     Ricotta and Chive Cloud Pancakes 42

     Mushroom and Spinach Frittata 42

     Almond and Coconut Flour Waffles 43

     Savory Yogurt Bowl with Roasted Veggies 43

     Zucchini Ricotta Pancakes 44

LUNCH RECIPES THAT NOURISH AND SATISFY 45

     Chilled Zucchini Noodle Salad with Flaked Salmon 46

     Hearty Turkey and White Bean Chili 46

     Asian Shrimp and Snow Pea Stir-Fry 47

     Spiced Lentil Soup with Spinach 47

     Chilled Avocado Soup with Lime and Cilantro 48

     Mediterranean Chickpea Salad 48

Turmeric Tofu and Kale Stir-Fry 49

Smoked Salmon and Cream Cheese Cucumber Rolls.. 49

Chilled Zucchini Ribbon Salad with Lemon and Herbs 50

Chilled Cucumber and Dill Soup... 50

Spicy Lentil and Carrot Soup 51

Apple Fennel Walnut Salad 51

Beetroot and Goat Cheese Arugula Salad 52

Cucumber Ribbon Salad with Feta and Mint 52

Hearty Beet and Barley Soup 53

Spicy Lentil and Spinach Soup 53

Avocado Chicken Salad with Lime and Cilantro 54

Thai Cucumber and Peanut Salad 54

Tuscan Bean Soup 55

Mushroom and Barley Stew.. 55

Spiced Lentil and Sweet Potato Stew.. 56

Cauliflower and Chickpea Masala 56

Lentil and Spinach Soup 57

Turkey and Barley Stew 57

Hearty Lentil Soup with Kale 58

DINNER RECIPES: DELIGHTS FOR DIABETICS 59

Cauliflower Rice Stir-Fry with Shrimp 60

Herbed Chicken and Zucchini Skillet 60

Beef and Broccoli Bowl with Cauliflower Mash 61

Sesame Ginger Salmon with Spinach 61

Zucchini and Bell Pepper Confetti Chicken 62

Creamy Turmeric Cauliflower Soup 62

Lemon Herb Grilled Salmon 63

Zucchini and Basil Pesto Stuffed Chicken 63

Turmeric Cauliflower Steaks with Tahini Drizzle 64

Grilled Salmon with Fennel and Orange Salad 64

Spicy Shrimp and Broccoli Stir-Fry 65

Zesty Lemon Herb Chicken... 65

Cauliflower Steak with Walnut Pesto 66

Spiced Rubbed Salmon with Cucumber Relish 66

Herbed Turkey and Spinach Meatballs 67

Zucchini Noodle Shrimp Scampi... 67

Lemon Herb Tilapia with Zucchini Ribbons 68

Spiced Chicken and Cauliflower Rice 68

Garlic Shrimp with Asparagus 69

Turmeric Ginger Salmon 69

Zucchini and Basil Frittata 70

Lemon Garlic Shrimp with Asparagus 70

Turmeric Chicken Stir-Fry... 71

Spiced Pork Tenderloin with Cauliflower Mash 71

Shrimp and Avocado Salad 72

SNACKS AND APPETIZERS: HEALTHY NIBBLES 73

Chia Seed and Coconut Yogurt Parfait 74

Spicy Roasted Chickpeas 74

Cucumber Roll-Ups with Hummus 75

Zesty Lime and Avocado Slices... 75

Chia Lemon Zest Bites 76

Savory Almond Flax Crackers 76

Cucumber Hummus Bites 77

Chili Lime Shrimp Cups 77

Mini Bell Pepper Nachos 78

Cucumber Avocado Rolls 78

Stuffed Mushrooms with Herbed Cheese 79

Grilled Zucchini Roll-Ups with Herbed Goat Cheese 79

Cucumber Cups with Smoked Salmon and Dill Cream 80

Shrimp and Avocado Cocktail Shooters 80

Cucumber Roll-Ups with Herbed Cream Cheese and Smoked Salmon 81

Cherry Tomatoes Stuffed with Goat Cheese and Herbs 81

Chia and Almond Butter Energy Balls 82

Peppered Turkey Jerky Strips 82

Savory Roasted Chickpeas 83

Spiced Pear Chips 83

Zesty Lemon Ricotta Bites 84

Smoky Paprika Chickpea Popcorn 84

Rosemary Beef Crostinis 85

Spicy Edamame Dip 85

Satisfying the SweetTooth: Dessert Recipes 86

Chia Chocolate Pudding 87

Almond Butter Fudge Squares 87

Coconut Lemon Bars 88

Avocado Cocoa Mousse 88

Zesty Lemon Ricotta Cheesecake 89

Spiced Avocado Chocolate Mousse 89

Almond Coconut Truffles 90

Berry Chia Pudding Parfait 90

Chia and Coconut Rice Pudding 91

Coconut and Almond No-Bake Cookies 91

Raspberry Chia Seed Pudding 92

Peanut Butter and Chocolate Hemp Squares 92

Lemon Cashew Date Bars 93

Almond Coconut Energy Balls 93

No-Bake Peanut Butter Oat Bars 94

Avocado Lime Cheesecake Cups 94

Cinnamon Walnut Fig Bites 95

Coconut & Almond Energy Balls 95

Kiwi Lime Sorbet 96

Baked Cinnamon Apple Chips 96

Raspberry Peach Gelatin Cups 97

Mango Coconut Frozen Yogurt 97

Chia and Raspberry Pudding 98

Peach Basil Sorbet 98

Blueberry Lime Drizzle 99

Kiwi Coconut Tartlets 99

A 49-Day Meal Plan 100

Beyond the Diet: Lifestyle and Mindset 103

Managing Stress and Emotional Eating 103

Community and Support Networks 104

Celebrating Milestones and Successes 106

Closing Reflections: Embracing a New Chapter 108

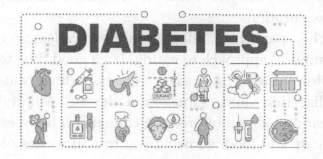

Welcome to a journey that begins at the crossroads of concern and hope—the unique challenge of managing diabetes post-50. It's here in these pages that we embrace the golden opportunity to seize control and truly thrive, transforming our diets and, by extension, our lives.

If you're like most people stepping into this chapter after a recent diagnosis, you might feel overwhelmed. Yet, coming to terms with diabetes or prediabetes in our later years, while admittedly daunting, can also unfold as a remarkably rewarding endeavour. It's a path paved not with restrictions but possibilities—where adapting to a healthier lifestyle gives rise to rediscovering the joy of food in its most nourishing form.

Managing diabetes is as much about filling your plate with what is beneficial as it is about understanding why these choices matter. Why does a low-carb, low-glycemic diet work wonders? How do these mindful decisions translate into stabilized blood sugar levels and, importantly, a vibrant, fuller life?

This book is crafted with the aim of demystifying the diet for diabetic management, making it not just accessible but enjoyable. Throughout these pages, I invite you to walk with me through practical, flavorful recipes that cater specifically to your needs while also delighting your palate. I'll guide you through understanding your body's responses, the profound impact of food on your wellbeing, and how, with a few adjustments, your diet can become your most potent ally in health management.

Furthermore, as we look ahead to the coming sections, we will delve into customized meal plans that simplify your journey, ensuring you're well-equipped to meet every day with confidence and zest. We'll explore together how each meal can become an opportunity to nurture yourself and connect with loved ones over dishes that everyone, regardless of their dietary needs, will find thoroughly satisfying.

So, let's begin with a hopeful heart and an open mind, ready to embark on this transformative endeavor where taste meets health, and every bite brings us closer to wellbeing.

EMBRACING CHANGE POST-50

Entering the stage of life beyond 50 brings its set of challenges and opportunities. While it may summon a certain nostalgia for youthful vigor and fewer concerns about chronic health conditions, it also heralds a time for personal growth and embracing change—particularly when managing diabetes or prediabetes. For many, turning 50 is not just a milestone but a wake-up call to take control of one's health more seriously than ever before.

Consider Julia, a vibrant 52-year-old who enjoyed a successful career and a bustling family life. Despite her energetic demeanor, she began experiencing fatigue and unexplainable bouts of thirst. A routine health check revealed her blood sugar levels were alarmingly high. This diagnosis was her unforeseen pivot to change. Rather than succumb to fear, Julia saw this as an opportunity to transform her life—beginning with her diet.

Diabetes, as daunting as it sounds, can be a gateway to profound life improvements. After

50, the body responds to food differently. Metabolic rates drop and the body's ability to process sugar diminishes. These biological changes necessitate a revised approach to eating—one that minimizes carbohydrates, favors low-glycemic foods, and regulates blood sugar levels.

Embarking on this dietary transition post-50 might seem overwhelming at first. However, the adjustment can be surprisingly seamless and rewarding. The key is to perceive this adjustment not as a restriction but as a journey towards culinary discovery and wellness. It's about replacing the sugar-laden and refined foods in your pantry with wholesome alternatives that are just as appetizing.

Adapting to dietary changes at this age also demands understanding of the role of different nutrients. Foods rich in fiber, such as leafy greens and whole grains, are essential as they slow the absorption of sugars, keeping blood glucose levels steady. Proteins become pivotal, not just for managing hunger but for aiding muscle repair and slowing carbohydrate absorption. Healthy fats from avocados, nuts, and olive oil should be embraced instead of feared, as they provide long-lasting energy and keep the heart healthy.

Moreover, beyond the plate, embracing change post-50 involves integrating physical activity into your routine. Walking, swimming, or yoga can not only aid in weight management but significantly impact blood sugar management, enhancing insulin sensitivity.

But let's not overlook the psychological adaptation to diabetes at this age. Turning 50 and facing a chronic illness can invoke frustrations and a sense of loss—mourning the freedom to eat without constraints or the burden of constant health monitoring. It's normal. Here is where building a supportive community—be it through online forums, local groups, or with friends and family—becomes invaluable. Sharing experiences and strategies not only alleviates the psychological burden but can also inspire delicious, healthful culinary explorations.

This period of adaptation also calls for a mindful approach to eating. It's a good time to slow down and savor meals, which aids digestion and satisfaction levels. Mindful eating helps reinforce the connection between body and food, allowing you to notice cues on satiety and enjoyment, better managing portions and cravings.

Practically speaking, regular monitoring of blood glucose levels will guide your dietary choices and adjustments. Over time, this routine won't just be about managing diabetes; it'll be about optimizing your health in a way that's tailored uniquely to you.

Embrace this change by exploring new foods and recipes. Discover the richness of flavors in diabetic-friendly spices like cinnamon and turmeric, which not only excite the palate but also offer health benefits, such as anti-inflammatory properties and aiding blood sugar control.

Remember, adapting your diet post-50 with a diabetes or prediabetes diagnosis is not a journey you have to embark on alone. Consult nutritionists, endocrinologists, and perhaps most importantly, connect with peers who are navigating similar paths. The shared stories of struggle and success are profoundly comforting and uplifting.

In adjusting your diet, you're not merely attempting to prevent the adverse effects of diabetes. You are setting the stage for a healthier, more energetic, and vibrant phase of life. It's about making peace with the changes while celebrating the variety and richness of foods that not only meet your nutritional needs but also delight your senses and bring joy to every meal.

Embracing change post-50, therefore, isn't just about managing a medical condition—it's about learning, experimenting, and finding joy in the new rhythms and patterns of a life lived well and healthfully. It's listening to your body, adjusting as needed, and always moving towards great health and happiness. Through this lens, each meal, each choice becomes an act of care and mindfulness, transforming the diabetic diet from a list of restrictions to a celebration of abundant, nourishing, and delectable foods.

UNDERSTANDING DIABETES IN YOUR GOLDEN YEARS

Breaching the golden years introduces us to a season of reflection, renewed priorities, and often, new health challenges to navigate. Among these, diabetes emerges as a prevalent counterpart for many, requiring us to glean a deeper understanding of how it interacts with the aging body and how it can be effectively managed.

Diabetes in your golden years is a complex dialogue between genetics, lifestyle choices, and how the body naturally transforms with age. The pancreas, which plays a crucial role in regulating blood sugar by producing insulin, might not function as efficiently as it once did. The result is often a diagnosis of Type 2 diabetes, where the body either resists the effects of insulin— a hormone necessary for sugar (glucose) to enter cells—or doesn't produce enough insulin to maintain a normal glucose level.

What many might not realize is that this isn't just about high blood sugar. The implications extend further, influencing everything from cardiovascular health to neurological well-being. This interconnected impact might seem daunting, but understanding is the first stepping stone toward effective management.

At this point in life, our bodies respond differently to food and exercise, and recovery from any form of injury or illness takes longer. Coupled with other age-related conditions, managing diabetes might feel like walking a tightrope. However, knowledge about how diabetes specifically affects your body during these years can transform that precarious walk into a steady stride.

For instance, it's essential to recognize symptoms often dismissed as 'signs of aging'. Increased thirst, frequent urination, fatigue, and blurred vision need careful attention and might require a consultation to rule out or confirm diabetes. Early detection plays a pivotal role in managing the disease more effectively and avoiding complications.

Understanding the glycemic index of foods becomes crucial, as blood sugar levels after meals impact overall control. Foods with a low glycemic index, such as non-starchy vegetables and whole grains, help maintain steady glucose levels. It's not merely about cutting out sugar but about knowing which carbohydrates provide sustained energy without significant glucose spikes.

In conjunction with dietary management, comprehending the physiological changes that affect metabolism helps tailor not just what you eat but also how you eat. Smaller, more frequent meals may be advantageous compared to the traditional three meals a day, aiding in more stable blood sugar levels throughout the day.

Age also affects how the body processes medication, including insulin. Those new to diabetes management might discover that their sensitivity to insulin changes, necessitating adjustments in dosages. Regular consultations with healthcare providers can lead to effective medication regimens that cater specifically to the older body's needs.

Moreover, aging impacts not just the body but also the mind. Mental health is paramount, as feelings of isolation or depression can accompany the lifestyle adjustments required by diabetes management. Engaging with community support groups, whether locally or online, provides emotional sustenance, which is just as crucial as dietary management.

Monitoring becomes a critical routine. Frequent blood glucose checks and regular visits to your healthcare provider help keep tabs on the progress and effectiveness of your diabetes management strategy. In the digital age, numerous apps and tools can help track your health data and provide insights that lead to informed decisions about your health.

Besides the nuts and bolts of managing blood sugar, there's a broader narrative to consider—your quality of life. Diabetes doesn't define your golden years; it simply integrates into a broader health management framework that includes enjoying life. Pursuing hobbies, connecting with friends and family, and traveling can all be part of your life with the right strategies in place.

As we dive deeper into the later chapters of this book, we will explore specific dietary strategies, but it's important to remember that a holistic approach considers all aspects of well-being. Managing diabetes in your golden years holds challenges, but with understanding, these challenges can be navigated successfully.

Embracing this season of your life with a proactive and informed stance on diabetes doesn't just add years to your life; it adds life to your years, enabling you to enjoy this rich period with vigor, peace, and fulfillment. Armed with knowledge and supported by a community, the journey through diabetes management can lead to a pathway of profound personal growth and well-being.

THE POWER OF DIET IN DIABETES MANAGEMENT

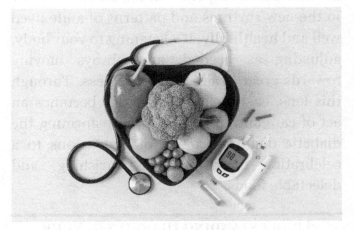

Imagine standing at the helm of a ship, navigating through misty waters; your compass is your diet, and your destination is optimal health management in the face of diabetes. The food choices you make can profoundly influence your journey, impacting everything from your daily energy levels to long-term disease outcomes. As we delve into understanding the powerful role that diet plays in diabetes management, it becomes clear that what you eat doesn't just fill your stomach—it can steer your health in lifeline directions.

Diabetes management has long been rooted in pharmaceuticals, examining what medicines can stabilize or improve conditions. However, emerging research underscores a crucial complementary strategy that requires just as much focus and finesse: dietary management. At its core, this involves understanding the types of foods, their composition, and their timing, which can collectively influence blood glucose levels and the body's overall response to insulin.

For someone managing diabetes, every meal represents a critical decision point that can either stabilize or destabilize blood sugar. Carbohydrates demand particular attention; they have a direct impact on blood glucose levels. However, the key isn't to eliminate carbs completely but to choose them wisely. Complex carbohydrates with low glycemic indices—such as whole grains, legumes, and most vegetables—digest more slowly, causing a gradual rise in blood sugar levels rather than a spike.

While carbohydrates often capture the spotlight in discussions about diabetes diet management, proteins and fats hold their pivotal roles. Proteins are essential not only for muscle repair and growth but also for blood sugar regulation. They help slow the absorption of glucose into the bloodstream, providing a steadier source of energy without the peaks and troughs. Similarly, healthy fats from sources like avocados, nuts, and olive oil contribute to satiety and support cellular function without directly spiking blood glucose.

The timing of meals can also play a critical role. Regular, balanced meals can prevent the highs and lows of blood glucose levels, stabilizing them throughout the day. This is particularly important for those on insulin or other medications that lower blood sugar, as it can help prevent the dangerous dips that occur when meals are skipped or delayed.

Beyond macronutrients, the dietary pattern overall matters significantly. The Mediterranean diet, for example, has been shown through various studies to be beneficial in managing diabetes due to its emphasis on whole foods, lean proteins, healthy fats, and an abundance of fresh produce. Diets rich in fiber are particularly effective, as fiber slows glucose absorption and improves insulin sensitivity.

Yet, managing diabetes isn't just about adhering to specific dietary rules—it's also about understanding how food behaves in your body and using that knowledge to tailor your diet. It's about making empowered and informed choices that not only cater to taste but also nurture your body's needs.

Diabetes education often highlights what not to eat, which can lead to a restrictive mindset. A more empowering approach focuses on what you can eat. This transformative view not only shifts one's emotional and psychological relationship with food but also opens up a spectrum of foods that enhance both health and palate satisfaction. It encourages people to explore a variety of nutrient-dense foods and to experiment with new recipes and flavors that align with a healthful eating plan, turning dietary management into a creative, enjoyable, and sustainable practice.

Monitoring how different foods affect blood sugar levels is also crucial. Self-monitoring of blood glucose (SMBG) can aid individuals in understanding their responses to various foods and refine their diet for optimal control over their condition. This practice of noting and adjusting accordingly can make the difference between a restrictive diabetic life and a flexible, health-oriented lifestyle.

One of the most inspiring aspects of dietary management is its potential to recover not just physical health but the joy of eating as well. While diabetes might narrow some food choices, it opens a range of culinary roads that might not have been explored otherwise. From experimenting with herbs and spices to replace salt or sugar to discovering local, seasonal vegetables that fill the plate with color and nutrients, each meal can be an exploration of discovery.

In essence, navigating diabetes effectively involves not just reacting to the condition with medication but actively managing it through thoughtful, well-informed food choices. Eating well can become both an art and a science where you are the most intrinsic part in the management of your health. As you adjust to this approach, embracing the full power of a tailored diet is not just about preventing complications—it's a steady commitment to thriving despite diabetes. Armed with knowledge and positive strategies, the journey ahead in your golden years can be navigated successfully with confidence and gusto.

SETTING REALISTIC GOALS

Embarking on the path of managing diabetes effectively, especially post-50, is akin to preparing for a rewarding journey. It's essential not just to know the destination but also to set realistic, achievable milestones that motivate and guide you. Setting realistic goals is at the heart of diabetes management—goals that challenge yet support you, pushing you towards optimal health while ensuring the journey is manageable and encouraging.

When you first receive a diagnosis of diabetes or are looking to tighten your control over it, the natural response is often one of drastic measures—overhauling your diet completely, exercising strenuously, or radically shifting your lifestyle overnight. However, experience and wisdom indicate that the most profound and lasting changes are those that are introduced gradually and with consideration.

The first step in setting these realistic goals is understanding exactly where you are in your health journey and where you want to be. This involves a detailed assessment—often with the help of healthcare professionals—of your current health metrics like blood glucose levels, HbA1c, cholesterol, blood pressure, and body weight. These figures provide a baseline from which progress can be measured.

From here, we move into goal-setting, grounded in the SMART criteria—specific, measurable, achievable, relevant, and time-bound. Consider a goal like "I want to improve my diet to better manage my diabetes." While its intention is good, it's vague and offers no roadmap for success or measurement. A SMART version of this goal might be, "I will limit my intake of processed carbohydrates to less than 90 grams per day and include at least two servings of vegetables in my meals, four days a week for the next three months." This goal isn't just precise; it's also incremental and measurable.

Each person's goals will differ, shaped by their unique life circumstances, metabolic health, and personal preferences. For some, weight loss might be a prioritized goal if it significantly impacts blood glucose control. For others, enhancing physical activity might be the focus, starting perhaps with a daily walk that eventually evolves into more varied and challenging exercise routines.

Realistic goal setting also involves anticipating and strategizing around potential barriers. Life doesn't pause while we pursue health management. Family commitments, work stresses, and social events will continue, and planning for ways to incorporate your health goals into these realities is crucial. For example, if family meals are a potential challenge due to dietary preferences differing from your diabetes-friendly needs, a realistic goal might be to craft a weekly dinner menu that includes options everyone can enjoy without derailing your management efforts.

An essential aspect of setting and achieving goals is tracking and accountability. Maintaining a journal or using a digital app to track food intake, exercise, and glucose levels can provide invaluable feedback and a tangible sense of progression. Regular check-ins with a diabetes educator or a dietitian not only offer professional insights but also reinforce commitment and can adjust goals as needed ensuring they remain realistic and attainable.

Moreover, setting realistic goals also means allowing for flexibility and forgiveness. There will be days when goals are not met, and that's okay. The journey to managing diabetes is marked not by perfection but by consistent effort and the ability to return to set routines after temporary setbacks.

Reflecting periodically on your accomplishments boosts morale and provides a clearer vision for the steps ahead. Celebrate successes, no matter how small they may seem—each is a step towards a healthier state. Whether it's noticing an improvement in your daily blood sugar levels, fitting into an old pair of pants, or simply feeling more energetic and healthier, acknowledgment of these victories can fuel motivation for continued effort.

Ultimately, the art of setting realistic goals in diabetes management is an ongoing process of calibration. It not only involves meticulous planning and proactive adjustments based on real-life feedback but also nurtures a positive mindset that cherishes progress in any form. By setting achievable targets, the journey through diabetes management becomes less daunting and more of a structured challenge, where each small victory accumulates into significant health and wellbeing advancements.

As you continue to set and refine your goals, remember that this journey is uniquely yours. Your targets, strategies, and paces are yours to define. With each step, you gain a deeper understanding of your body's responses, and each milestone reached is a testament to your commitment to living well with diabetes. Embrace this path with resilience and optimism, and let each realistic goal set bring you closer to the health and vitality you seek in your golden years.

NAVIGATING THE DIABETIC DIET LANDSCAPE

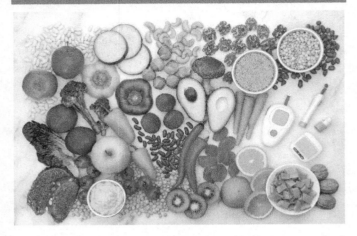

Diving into the world of diabetic diets can feel like navigating a maze with its twists and turns, especially after you've crossed the golden mark of fifty. The foods you once loved might now seem like forbidden fruits, and the sheer volume of dietary advice can be overwhelming. However, understanding how to balance your meals isn't just about avoiding certain foods—it's about rediscovering the joy in eating and turning nourishment into a tool for wellness.

Imagine you're setting sail on a serene journey, not battling a tempest. Here in this chapter, we will explore this tranquil voyage—the calm waters of diabetic dietary management where stormy seas and rocky shores appear far less daunting. Let's consider each meal an opportunity—a chance to fuel your body in ways that stabilize your blood sugar and enhance your overall health.

Through these pages, we'll delve into what makes a diet effective for managing diabetes past age fifty. It's not solely about counting carbs or avoiding sugar. It's about understanding the nutritional value of foods, how they interact with your body, and how they can be combined to not only satisfy your appetite but also manage your condition. We will look at how diabetes affects your body differently as you age and adjust our sails accordingly.

Picture this: each recipe and each meal plan is a compass guiding you through a landscape dotted with rich flavors and ingredients that cater to your health needs without sacrificing taste. With each chapter, we shall decode the myths surrounding diabetic eating, unearth hidden sugars that sneak into the most unsuspecting of foods, and learn how to create a balanced plate that keeps both your palate and your blood sugar in check.

Navigating this diet isn't about stringent restrictions that darken your dining experience; it's about making informed choices that brighten your life. Together, we'll find that sweet spot—where managing diabetes feels not just manageable, but enjoyable. Let's savor each dish, relish each bite, and turn dietary management into a flavorful feast for the senses.

DECIPHERING NUTRITIONAL NEEDS AFTER 50

As we voyage past the age of 50, our bodies begin to narrate a different story. This new chapter, often marked by a slowing metabolism and changing nutritional needs, calls for a fresh approach to eating—especially for those managing diabetes. The metabolism naturally slows, the body's ability to process sugar changes, and suddenly, managing dietary needs becomes a critical narrative in the story of our health.

Understanding these changes is essential in crafting a diet that not only pleases the palate but also supports our unique health needs. After 50, the body requires fewer calories, yet the demand for certain nutrients increases, often making the balance between 'eating well' and 'eating right' a delicate dance.

The Metabolic Shift

Firstly, let's address the elephant in the room—metabolism. Why does it slow down? As we age, our muscle mass naturally decreases. Since muscle burns more calories than fat, this reduction slows our metabolism, necessitating fewer calories to maintain the same weight. However, reducing calorie intake doesn't mean sacrificing nutritional richness. The key is to select foods densely packed with nutrients yet moderate in calories. This means embracing vibrant vegetables, lean proteins, whole grains, and healthy fats, which provide satiety and support blood sugar control.

Calcium and Bone Health

Then there's the matter of bone density. After 50, the risk of osteoporosis begins to climb, especially among women post-menopause. Calcium, vital for bone health, should be a starring character in your dietary lineup. However, balancing calcium intake is more nuanced for those with diabetes, as large quantities of some calcium-rich foods (like high-fat dairy products) can be laden with unhealthy fats. Instead, a focus on low-fat dairy options, fortified plant milks, and leafy greens can help maintain bone health without compromising blood glucose levels.

Fiber's Leading Role

Fiber deserves a leading role in your diet after 50. Not only does it aid digestion, but it also plays a significant part in controlling blood sugar levels and aiding in weight management—crucial for those managing diabetes. Foods high in fiber such as lentils, beans, vegetables, and whole grains should be regular heroes on your plate. However, integrating fiber must be a gradual narrative in your diet to prevent digestive distress.

Protein and Muscle Maintenance

As the story of our body's muscle mass presents a bit of a downturn, protein needs a spotlight. Adequate protein intake supports muscle health, counters muscle loss, and by virtue of its slower digestion (compared to carbohydrates), assists in managing blood glucose levels. However, the selection of protein sources should lean on lean meats, fish, plant-based alternatives, and poultry, stepping away from excessive red meat consumption which can lead to other health complications.

Vitamins and Minerals

Another subplot in our nutritional narrative after 50 is the absorption of vitamins and minerals. Vitamin B12, which helps keep nerve and blood cells healthy, becomes harder to absorb with age. The plot thickens for many with diabetes as metformin, a common diabetes medication, further complicates B12 absorption. Thus, fortified foods or supplements might become necessary characters in our diet.

Similarly, Vitamin D, essential not only for bone health but also potentially for blood sugar control, often requires supplementation due to decreased skin synthesis with age and limited dietary sources.

Managing Blood Pressure

Salt — once perhaps a minor character in our younger days—takes on a more antagonistic role after 50, especially for those with hypertension, which often accompanies diabetes. Lowering sodium intake by avoiding processed foods and seasoning with herbs and spices can drastically improve this subplot.

Hydration

Often overlooked yet crucial is the role of water. Hydration plays a critical part in overall health and aids in kidney function — pivotal for those managing diabetes as the risk of kidney issues escalates with age. Ensuring a consistent hydration habit helps maintain kidney health and supports all bodily functions.

Balancing Act

So how do you balance this ensemble cast of nutrients? It starts with mindful eating—

listening to your body's cues and understanding the effects foods have on your blood sugar levels. Regular meals, portion control, and a diverse plate are fundamental practices. But this isn't about stringent dietary limitations; it's about creating a colorful, varied diet that includes all food groups, providing both pleasure and nutritional benefits.

Uncharted Waters

Embarking on this journey requires tuning into your body's signals and adapting as your needs evolve. Regular discussions with healthcare providers can guide adjustments in your diet, ensuring it continually aligns with your health status, lifestyle, and, importantly, your diabetes management plan.

Understanding and adapting to your nutritional needs after 50 is not just about crossing a treacherous sea of restrictions; it's about navigating a river of opportunities, each meal a chance to nourish both body and soul, aligning the pleasures of eating with the needs of living. This journey is not one of scarcity but abundance, where each choice brings you closer to harmony between pleasure and health.

THE DO'S AND DON'TS: FOODS FOR DIABETES

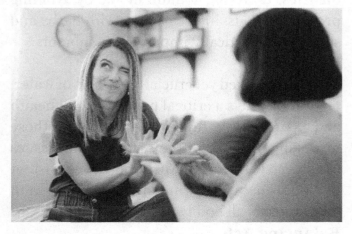

Embarking on a dietary journey with diabetes can sometimes feel like navigating a culinary maze without a map. The landscape is dotted with foods masked as friends or foes, making each meal choice seem like a crucial turn. But fear not; understanding the 'dos and don'ts' in your diet is akin to discovering safe passages through a potentially treacherous terrain—turning daily meals from confusing choices into opportunities for enhancing your health.

The Trustworthy Paths: The Dos

The 'dos' in your diabetic diet are foods that work in favor to manage your blood sugar, enhance your overall health, and make every meal a celebration of flavor, without the worry.

Fiber-Filled Champions: Start by embracing whole grains like barley, quinoa, and whole oats. These aren't just hearty and filling; they have a gentler effect on your blood glucose levels compared to their refined counterparts. Then, there are the vegetables—towering pillars of nutrition. Non-starchy varieties such as leafy greens, peppers, and broccoli are true heroes, hosting an array of vitamins, minerals, and precious fiber.

Lean Proteins: Whether it's chicken breast, fish like salmon and tuna rich in omega-3 fatty acids, or plant-based sources like lentils and chickpeas, lean proteins are vital. They provide the building blocks for your body without excessive fat or calories, hence not weighing down your blood sugar levels.

Healthy Fats: Think of avocados, nuts, seeds, and olive oil as your allies that march at your side. These sources of monounsaturated and polyunsaturated fats not only support heart health—a concern for many with diabetes—but also enhance satiety, helping curb unhealthy snacking.

The Wise Additions: Season your dishes with herbs and spices instead of salt, enriching your food with flavors while dodging the blood pressure pitfalls. Also, consider the power of hydration—water herbs like mint or cucumber to add a refreshing twist, encouraging better hydration habits without added sugars.

The Misleading Detours: The Don'ts

The 'don'ts'—often tempting and indulgent—are the foods likely to spike your blood glucose levels and sabotage your health goals if consumed indiscriminately.

Sugary Sirens: Regular sodas, candies, and desserts rich in refined sugars are as tempting as they are treacherous. They lead to swift spikes in blood sugar and can be addictive, making it difficult to control portions and cravings.

Refined Grains: White bread, pasta made from white flour, and other heavily processed grains act almost like sugary foods in your body. They break down quickly, catapulting your glucose levels to unwelcome peaks.

High-Sodium Traps: Processed foods not only harbor unhealthy fats and additives but are typically laden with sodium. Excessive salt intake can raise blood pressure, an unwanted companion for cardiovascular health.

Saturated and Trans Fats: These fats, commonly found in butter, margarine, and fried foods, contribute to heart disease risk and may affect insulin resistance. A tip here is to cook with methods that require less or no fat, like baking, grilling, or steaming.

Navigating the landscape of diabetic eating isn't just about avoiding the 'don'ts' but transforming the 'dos' into daily habits that enhance your health without leaving you feeling deprived. It's about making each meal a step towards wellness.

Crafting Your Culinary Map

As you compile your safe travel guide through diabetes management, consider every meal an exploration. Fill half of your plate with non-starchy vegetables, a quarter with lean protein, and the other quarter with a portion of whole grains or a starchy vegetable. This not only visually simplifies your meal planning but ensures balance in every bite.

The real art lies in altering routes according to your diary of blood sugar levels. Sometimes, a path thought safe might need reassessment. The flexibility to adjust your course based on ongoing feedback from your body is crucial.

Making Peace with the Journey

Remember, managing diabetes through diet is not a punitive measure—it's a transformative journey meant to enrich your life with wholesome and delightful eating experiences. The 'dos and don'ts' are not just rules but symbols of a balanced, enjoyable feeding philosophy that nourishes both body and spirit. Lastly, partner with your healthcare team—use their expertise as a compass to guide your dietary decisions. This collaborative approach ensures that your diabetic diet map is both personalized and effective, turning the act of eating into a joyful, health-giving part of your life. Every meal then becomes an opportunity to nurture your body, delight your palate, and manage your diabetes with confidence and grace.

BALANCING BLOOD SUGAR WITH SMART EATING

In the journey of managing diabetes, particularly post-50, balancing blood sugar becomes a central narrative of daily eating habits. It's like setting the sails of a ship; too much wind and you're off course, too little and you're adrift. Intelligent meal planning—not just what you eat, but how and when you eat—ensures that your metabolism doesn't swing too dramatically in either direction.

Understanding the Glycemic Symphony

The concept of glycemic control is akin to conducting an orchestra. Each food plays a different instrument, contributing its unique sound to the overall blood sugar levels in your body. Foods with a high glycemic index play loud, fast tunes, causing your blood sugars to spike quickly. On the other hand, low glycemic index foods deliver a smoother, more sustained sound, keeping your blood sugars stable.

Harmonizing Your Meals

Picture your meal as a balanced musical ensemble. Start with a strong base of fiber-rich vegetables and whole grains—these are your cellos and double basses, providing deep, sustained tones that keep the melody of your metabolism harmonious. Add in lean proteins—your violins, offering balance and texture to the composition. Finally, incorporate healthy fats, the harps of your nutritional orchestra, enriching the melody without overwhelming it.

Timing is Key

Just as important as what you eat is when you eat. The body metabolizes food differently throughout the day, and eating regularly helps avoid the highs and lows that can feel like metabolic whiplash. Small, frequent meals—like movements in a symphony—can keep the body's metabolic rate steady and efficient. Skipping meals, on the other hand, can send your body into an emergency mode, increasing insulin resistance and blood sugar levels in the long term.

The Role of Hydration

Amidst fine-tuning macronutrients, let's not overlook the fluid that cleanses the palate between dishes—water. Hydrating regularly helps moderate blood sugar levels, aids digestion, and ensures that nutrients circulate efficiently throughout your body. Consider it the acoustic insulation in your concert hall, essential but often unnoticed.

Beyond Just Sugar

While managing intake of obvious sugars is crucial, understanding insulin function and resistance is vital. Every bite activates a complex dance of hormonal and metabolic responses. Foods that might seem benign or even healthy can provoke unexpected responses in your body, particularly if insulin resistance is part of your narrative.

The Danger of Hidden Sugars

Navigating the hidden sugars in processed foods is like uncovering disguised traps in a treasure hunt. These sugars, often masquerading under names like fructose or sucrose, can make managing diabetes an unexpected challenge. They pop up in sauces, breads, and even foods promoted as "health foods," playing a discordant note in your blood sugar levels.

Sensible Snacking

Snacks are not just intermissions; they can be pivotal in maintaining rhythm in your blood sugar levels. Strategic snacking, especially on foods rich in protein and fiber, can act as miniature metabolic concerts throughout the day, maintaining your energy and keeping hunger at bay without causing sugar spikes.

Psychological Balance and Smart Eating

The dialogue between mind and stomach is profound. Stress, anxiety, and even boredom often send us to the kitchen, seeking comfort in food. Balancing blood sugar is not only about the physical act of eating but also managing these emotional cues that can disrupt our nutritional harmony.

The Empowerment of Knowledge

Understanding the impact of what you eat, how foods interact, and how they transform within your body empowers you to make smarter choices. Knowledge, in this context, acts like sheet music to a novice musician, providing guidance and confidence to turn individual notes into melodious health outcomes.

Crafting a Personalized Eating Score

Just as every musician tweaks their instrument to play its sweetest tune, so too must individuals with diabetes fine-tune their diets. What works for one person might not work for another, and factors like age, activity level, and additional health issues play significant roles in each person's dietary needs.

Closing Thoughts on Balanced Eating

As we traverse through the landscape of diabetes management, remember that smart eating is a journey, not a destination. It's a continuous process of learning and adjusting, akin to perfecting a musical piece. Balancing blood sugar with smart eating involves harmonizing all aspects of your life—from diet to exercise, from stress management to regular medical checkups—creating a symphony of health that supports not just managing diabetes but thriving with it.

In essence, the mastery of balancing blood sugar doesn't come from strict adherence to rigid rules but from understanding the broader metabolic melody and how different foods, habits, and timings contribute to its harmony. This knowledge not only ensures dietary compliance but enriches your life, making each meal a note in the symphony of your well-being.

UNEARTHING HIDDEN SUGARS IN EVERYDAY FOODS

Navigating the diabetic diet often feels akin to being a detective in a culinary mystery, where sugars cunningly hide in the most unanticipated of places. These hidden sugars, lurking within seemingly innocent everyday foods, pose significant challenges for those striving to manage their blood sugar levels and overall health. Uncovering them is not just a matter of keen observation but an act of safeguarding one's well-being.

The Masquerade of Sugars

At first glance, many foods may appear diabetes-friendly. However, upon closer inspection, labels reveal a different story—a tale of hidden sugars disguised under various aliases. These sugars are adept at evasion, listed on ingredient labels as maltose, fructose, dextrose, and more than fifty other names that might easily be overlooked by the untrained eye.

Breakfast: A Sugary Start?

Consider the morning routine, often believed to be healthy—a bowl of cereal, some flavored yogurt, a glass of juice. These staples, though seemingly benign, can sometimes contain as much sugar as a dessert. Many breakfast cereals, even those branded as 'whole-grain' or 'fiber-rich', can be high in added sugars. Flavored yogurts, too, often have a sugar content comparable to ice cream. And fruit juices, even 100% fruit varieties, concentrate sugars while lacking the fiber of their whole fruit counterparts, leading to faster rises in blood glucose.

The Sauces and Dressings Dilemma

Venture further into the average kitchen pantry, and one finds shelves lined with sauces, dressings, and condiments. From ketchup to barbecue sauce, teriyaki to salad dressings, these convenient flavor boosters can be riddled with sugars. A mere tablespoon of ketchup may contain around a teaspoon of sugar. Thus, a seemingly health-conscious choice of a salad can inadvertently become a high-sugar meal due to its dressing.

Health Foods: Not Always Healthy

The quest continues with foods marketed as 'health foods'—granola bars, smoothies, protein shakes, and energy bars. These products, often aimed at those pursuing a healthy lifestyle, can be surprisingly sugar-packed. Take the example of granola bars, perceived as a healthy snack or quick breakfast alternative. Despite their health halo, many are held together with syrups and binding agents rich in sugars. Similarly, store-bought smoothies and protein shakes might boast fruit and other healthy ingredients but are frequently sweetened with added sugars for taste enhancement.

The Bread Basket

It's not just the overtly sweet foods; starchy foods like bread can also contribute to the hidden sugar trap. While not high in sugars themselves, the types of carbohydrates present in many processed bread can lead to similar glycemic responses as outright sugar. This is due to the body rapidly converting these refined carbs into glucose.

Decoding Labels: A Tool for Transparency

Averting the pitfalls of hidden sugars necessitates becoming fluent in the language of food labeling. Translating a food label to identify sugar content involves more than scanning for the word 'sugar'—it demands an understanding of all its disguises. Moreover, it's important to look beyond the grams of sugar and assess the list of ingredients, noting their order of appearance, which signifies their proportion in the product.

Portion Sizes: An Accomplice to Sugar

Another element in the hidden sugar puzzle is portion size. Packaging can mislead with 'serving sizes' that are much smaller than the typical amount one might consume. For example, a drink bottle that appears designed for one might list nutritional contents for two servings, doubling the expected sugar intake if one isn't vigilant.

Alternative Sweeteners: A Bittersweet Solution

While alternative sweeteners like stevia, xylitol, and erythritol offer sweetness without traditional sugars, they should be used judiciously. Understanding their effects on your blood sugar and overall health requires careful consideration and perhaps consultation with a health professional, as reactions can vary widely among individuals with diabetes.

Smart Shopping and Eating: Keys to Unlocking Health

Unmasking hidden sugars goes beyond scrutiny—it's about making informed choices. Choose whole, unprocessed foods when possible, as these naturally contain minimal to no added sugars. When purchasing processed items, opt for those labeled 'no added sugar' or with healthful sweeteners. Learn to appreciate the natural sweetness in foods, such as fruits and vegetables, and spice up meals with herbs and spices instead of relying on sugary condiments.

A Journey of Discovery

Understanding hidden sugars isn't just about avoidance; it's a journey towards empowerment. By learning where sugars hide and how to avoid them, individuals with diabetes can take control of their diet, improve their health outcomes, and still enjoy a diverse and delicious diet. This journey doesn't just have a single destination but is a continual path of learning and adapting—one that leads to healthier habits and a fuller understanding of what it means to eat well with diabetes.

WELLNESS AND WHOLESOME INGREDIENTS

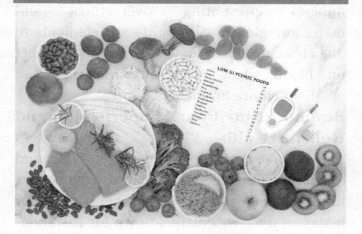

Welcome to a journey where health meets flavor right in your kitchen with essential, wholesome ingredients—a chapter dedicated to transforming your staple groceries into powerhouse meals that cater perfectly to your diabetic diet needs. In this part of our culinary adventure, we're focusing on the cornerstones that make up nourishing, diabetes-friendly meals, delving into superfoods, quality sourcing, and the enlightening world of food labels.

Think of your kitchen as a garden where every ingredient holds potential—each spice, vegetable, and protein is a tool to enhance not only taste but also your health. We often hear about 'superfoods,' a term that can sometimes seem daunting or exotic. Here, we'll break down exactly what makes an ingredient a "superfood" and how these can be both accessible and integral to managing your diabetes effectively after 50. From chia seeds throwing a punch of fiber into your breakfast smoothie to turmeric spicing up a low-carb stir-fry with its anti-inflammatory prowess, we'll explore how these heroes of the food world can be everyday staples rather than rarities.

But where do these ingredients come from? And how do we choose the best ones? The answers lie in understanding how to source and select high-quality ingredients. Whether it's choosing between organic or non-GMO, local or imported, the decisions can be overwhelming. However, by the end of this section, you'll be equipped with practical tips to make informed choices about the foods you bring into your home, ensuring they are not only delicious but also optimized for your health needs.

Furthermore, in an age where food labels can be more puzzling than helpful, gaining clarity on what terms like 'low-fat,' 'sugar-free,' and 'high in fiber' mean will empower you to make choices that align with your dietary goals. Each label tells a story about what's inside the packaging and understanding this narrative is key to managing your diabetes confidently.

By embarking on this informative path, you'll transform the way you view your pantry and refrigerator. This chapter is more than just about choosing ingredients; it's about making choices that respect your body's needs, allowing you to live vibrantly and healthily. Where every meal isn't just food, but a celebration of well-managed health and satisfying flavors.

SUPERFOODS FOR DIABETIC HEALTH

In the realm of managing diabetes—especially past the golden age of 50—incorporating superfoods into your diet can be a game-changer. These nutritional powerhouses pack a punch not only by adding rich flavors and textures to your meals but also by delivering substantial health benefits that particularly resonate with the needs of individuals managing diabetes or prediabetes. Understanding and harnessing the power of superfoods can transform daily nutrition from a mundane task into an exciting journey towards improved health.

Superfoods have earned their title due to their high density of nutrients. These include antioxidants, vitamins, and minerals, which are crucial for combating inflammation, enhancing immunity, and reducing blood sugar spikes—all significant concerns for diabetics.

The Balancing Act of Blood Sugar Levels

One primary concern for those managing diabetes is maintaining steady blood sugar levels. Foods high in fiber, such as leafy greens, berries, and legumes, play a pivotal role here. The magic in fiber lies in its ability to slow down the absorption of glucose into the bloodstream, thereby preventing the dramatic spikes and dips that can complicate diabetes management.

Antioxidants: Nature's Shield

Antioxidants are another critical component found abundantly in superfoods like blueberries, dark chocolate, and pecans. For someone with diabetes, these compounds are invaluable as they help reduce oxidative stress and inflammation, a common issue that can exacerbate diabetes complications. Foods rich in vitamin C, vitamin E, and selenium are not just good; they are essential in a diabetic's diet to aid in warding off cellular damage and supporting overall health.

Focusing on Fats: The Good Kind

In the discussion of diabetes management, the type of fat in one's diet cannot be overlooked. The health community once villainized all fats, but now we understand that healthy fats are exceptionally beneficial—avocados and nuts are stellar sources. They do not impact blood glucose levels and are thus an excellent energy source. Moreover, they help absorb fat-soluble vitamins and stabilize heart rhythms, which can be particularly advantageous as diabetes heightens cardiovascular risk.

Proteins: Building Blocks to Blood Sugar Control

Lean protein sources like fish rich in omega-3 fatty acids (such as salmon and sardines), skinless poultry, and tofu offer substantial benefits beyond just muscle repair and growth. They induce satiety, which helps in managing hunger, preventing overeating, and maintaining an ideal weight—key elements in diabetes care. Plus, they have minimal impact on blood sugar levels, making them an excellent choice for meal planning.

Beyond Nutrition: Superfoods and Holistic Health

The influence of superfoods extends beyond direct nutritional benefits; they also play a part in enhancing psychological well-being. For instance, dark chocolate, known for its mood-boosting properties, can elevate serotonin levels, contributing to better mental health. Knowing you're doing something good for your body also uplifts your spirit, reinforcing a positive mindset towards managing diabetes.

Practical Tips for Integrating Superfoods into Your Diet

Embracing superfoods doesn't mean revamping your entire pantry immediately; instead, gradually introduce these foods into your meals. Start by adding slices of avocado to your salad or swapping out your usual snack for a handful of almonds. Sprinkle some chia seeds or flaxseeds into your breakfast cereal or smoothie for a fiber-rich start to the day.

Consider revamping the oils in your kitchen too; replace some of the less healthy fats with olive oil or coconut oil, both reputed for their health benefits. These small changes can culminate in a significantly improved diet, aligning better with your health goals without sacrificing taste or satisfaction.

Incorporating superfoods into your diet when managing diabetes or prediabetes isn't just about following trends. It's about thoughtfully choosing ingredients that maximize your nutritional intake, fortify your body against the challenges of diabetes, and enhance your overall quality of life. Each meal becomes a step toward a more vibrant health narrative, where what you eat supports not just the body's requirements but also uplifts the spirit. In this light, superfoods are less of a dietary option and more of a lifestyle choice—an investment in a healthier, more joyful future.

SOURCING AND SELECTING QUALITY INGREDIENTS

Embarking on a journey to manage diabetes or prediabetes isn't just about adjusting what you eat; it's also profoundly connected to the quality and source of your ingredients. Choosing the right elements for your meals plays a pivotal role in managing your health and enhancing the flavors of your food. This narrative guides you through that selection process, demystifying terms and offering insights into making the healthiest choices possible, regardless of where you shop or dine. Imagine walking into a farmers' market: the fresh aromas, the vibrant colors, the sheer variety of natural foods. It's not just a feast for the senses; it's the ideal setting to begin selecting high-quality ingredients. But what makes an ingredient "high quality"? It's not just about organic labels—it's about how fresh the food is, how it was grown, and how far it travelled to get to your table.

Freshness First: Local Over Long-Haul

One of the first markers of quality is freshness. Fresh ingredients contain more nutrients, which are crucial for managing blood sugar levels and overall health. Locally sourced produce not just supports local economies but also tends to be fresher than its long-hauled counterparts. These foods haven't been stored for long periods or traveled thousands of miles, which often necessitates picking them before they have fully ripened, diminishing their nutritional profile.

The Organic Question: To Buy or Not to Buy?

The debate around organic foods is ever-present. Organic farming avoids the use of synthetic pesticides and fertilizers, genetically modified organisms (GMOs), and the routine use of antibiotics and hormones in livestock. For someone managing diabetes, the lack of pesticides means less risk of ingesting toxins that can affect insulin sensitivity and overall health.

However, organic food often comes with a higher price tag. It's essential to balance the benefits with your budget. A good strategy is to refer to environmental working groups like the EWG's Dirty Dozen™ list which details produce that typically harbors higher pesticide residues, making them ideal candidates for the organic aisle. Meanwhile, the Clean Fifteen™ can be purchased conventionally due to their low pesticide levels.

Understanding Labels: Transparency at Your Fingertips

Decoding labels is another key aspect of selecting quality ingredients. Terms like "all-natural" can be misleading, as they are not regulated by strict standards. Instead, look for labels that offer clarity about the product's origins and handling, such as "certified organic," "non-GMO," or "grass-fed." These labels entail that the food meets particular standards that might align better with your needs as a diabetic.

The Non-GMO Imperative

For many health-conscious shoppers, avoiding GMOs is a priority. The argument here extends beyond just health concerns; it includes environmental implications and personal preferences regarding agricultural practices. Non-GMO products ensure that you consume foods that are produced without genetic engineering, which some studies suggest might influence glucose intolerance and affect insulin regulation.

Grains, Nuts, and Legumes: Picking the Best

When it comes to grains, nuts, and legumes, the selection process might seem daunting. Opt for whole, unprocessed versions of these foods. Whole grains like quinoa, barley, and oats offer more fiber, helping to regulate blood sugar levels. With nuts, freshness and minimal processing (unsalted, unroasted) preserve their natural oils and nutrients that benefit heart health—a major concern for those with diabetes.

Meat and Fish: What to Look For

Selecting meat and fish also requires special consideration. Ideally, look for sustainably caught or responsibly farmed fish which ensures minimal exposure to contaminants like mercury and polychlorinated biphenyls (PCBs), which pose health risks. For poultry and meat, choose cuts from animals raised with good welfare standards and without the use of preventive antibiotics or added hormones. These practices affect the meat's quality and can have implications for your health.

Dairy Deliberations: Full Fat, Low Fat, No Fat?

The full-fat versus low-fat debate in dairy products is particularly relevant. Full-fat dairy has been shown in some studies to aid in weight control and promote heart health, which is vital for diabetes management. However, moderation is critical. Opting for products like yogurt, cheese, and milk from grass-fed cows can enhance their fatty acid profile, making them healthier for your diabetic diet.

As you embark on your next shopping trip, remember that selecting quality ingredients isn't just about enhancing the flavor of your meals—it's about investing in your health and taking control of your diabetes in a way that aligns with nature and science. Each choice you make at the grocery store is a step toward a healthier, more vibrant you.

THE ROLE OF ORGANIC AND NON-GMO FOODS

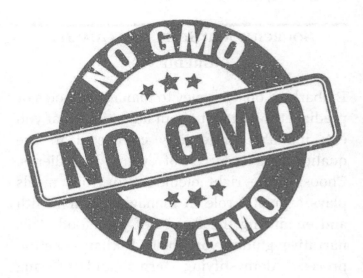

In the quest for a healthier lifestyle, especially post-diagnosis of diabetes or prediabetes, understanding the role of organic and non-GMO foods can be akin to unraveling a finely knitted sweater. Every thread counts, and each decision about what to put on your plate holds potential impacts for your long-term health. This chapter explores the significance of these food classifications and how they fit into a diabetes management plan centered around wholesome nutrition.

Organic Foods: Beyond the Buzzword

The term "organic" refers to how agricultural products are grown and processed. For a food to be certified organic, stringent guidelines must be followed that restrict the use of synthetic pesticides, fertilizers, and genetically modified organisms (GMOs). Livestock raised for organic meat, dairy, and eggs must have access to the outdoors and be fed organic feed without the routine use of antibiotics or growth hormones.

These standards mirror a growing awareness and preference for food production methods that are believed to be safer and more sustainable, but for those with diabetes, the conversation digs deeper. Organic foods often have lower pesticide residues, which is crucial since some pesticides can interfere with insulin regulation and increase the burden on the liver, complicating the body's natural balance of hormones and glucose levels.

Nutritional Considerations: Is Organic Really Better?

Studies have shown that organic foods can have higher nutritional value in terms of antioxidants and certain vitamins and minerals. Antioxidants play a significant role for those with diabetes by reducing oxidative stress, which is linked to insulin resistance. Foods such as berries, leafy greens, and nuts are often recommended in heightened quantities in diabetic diets, and their organic versions can provide an added advantage, offering purer forms of these crucial nutrients without the chemical additives.

Non-GMO: Understanding the Genetic Blueprint

GMOs are organisms that have had their DNA altered in ways that do not occur naturally. The primary goal behind their development was to increase crop yield and resistance to pests and diseases. However, the long-term health impacts of consuming GMO foods are still a subject of on-going research and debate.

For individuals managing diabetes, the focus on non-GMO foods often stems from concerns about the unknown effects these modifications might have on sugar metabolism and overall endocrine function. Choosing non-GMO foods is considered a proactive approach to eliminate potential risks, especially when the interaction of such altered foods with diabetes isn't fully understood.

Practical Tips for Incorporating Organic and Non-GMO Foods

Navigating a grocery store's organic and non-GMO offerings can be overwhelming. Here are a few practical strategies to integrate these foods into your diet thoughtfully:

1. **Start with the Dirty Dozen and Clean Fifteen**: These lists, published annually, help prioritize which fruits and vegetables to buy organic based on pesticide residue levels.
2. **Read Labels Carefully**: Certification labels for organic and non-GMO products include USDA Organic and Non-GMO Project Verified. These labels ensure that the food complies with national standards for organic and non-GMO farming.
3. **Local Markets and Farms**: Purchasing your produce, meats, and dairy at local farmer's markets can provide access to organic and non-GMO products while supporting local agriculture.
4. **Grow Your Own**: Starting a garden with organic seeds is another way to ensure you are consuming fresh, nutrient-rich foods without the worry of harmful additives.

Economic Considerations

While the benefits of choosing organic and non-GMO products align closely with the dietary needs of individuals with diabetes, cost can be a significant barrier. Organic foods are often more expensive due to more labor-intensive agricultural practices and lower yields. However, investing in health can be seen as a proactive measure against potential medical expenses associated with diabetes complications down the line. Budget-conscious approaches, such as buying in bulk, choosing frozen organic produce, or focusing on the Dirty Dozen, can mitigate some of these costs.

In conclusion, integrating organic and non-GMO foods into a diabetic diet isn't merely about following a trend but about making informed choices for long-term health management. These choices impact not only personal health but also broader environmental and ethical issues, knitting together personal well-being with global consciousness. In the journey of managing diabetes, every bite counts, and understanding what makes each bite beneficial can lead to a more sustainable, healthful, and satisfying lifestyle.

UNDERSTANDING FOOD LABELS AND CLAIMS

Navigating the world of food labels and claims can often feel like deciphering a secret code—particularly for those managing health conditions like diabetes, where every ingredient plays a vital role. Understanding what these labels represent is akin to learning a new language—one that speaks directly to the quality and safety of your food.

At first glance, labels might present a dizzying array of terms—organic, free-range, non-GMO, no added sugars, low-carb—and each term carries its own weight and relevance. The key to turning these labels from confusing to empowering lies in mastering the ability to interpret them accurately, ensuring they align with your dietary needs.

Breaking Down 'Nutrition Facts'

Every packaged food in a grocery store comes adorned with a "Nutrition Facts" label, mandated by various health authorities around the globe. This label is your first stop to understanding the nutritional content of the food. It outlines key components—calories, fats, carbohydrates, proteins, and other essential nutrients. For those managing diabetes, particular attention should be paid to the sections detailing total carbohydrates, including dietary fiber, sugars, and added sugars. Understanding these numbers is crucial in planning meals that maintain blood glucose levels within target ranges.

Beyond Nutrition: Ingredient Lists

While the Nutrition Facts panel tells you about quantities, the ingredient list tells you about quality. Ingredients are listed in order of quantity, from highest to lowest. This section is particularly critical for spotting hidden sugars, unhealthy fats, and potential allergens. Terms like "dextrose," "fructose," and "syrup" can often fly under the radar as sugar sources. For a person with diabetes, recognizing these hidden sugars is essential to avoid unintentional spikes in blood sugar.

Deciphering Health Claims

Food labels are also often adorned with various health claims. These can range from "light" or "lite" to "heart-healthy" or "lowers cholesterol." These terms are regulated by health authorities and they usually mean that the product has met specific criteria to qualify for these claims. However, it's important to read such labels with a critical eye—especially claims like "low-fat" and "fat-free," as these products might have added sugars to compensate for taste, which can be detrimental to blood sugar management.

Organic and Non-GMO Labels

As previously discussed, organic and non-GMO labels signify products made without the use of synthetic pesticides, genetic modification, and certain additives. These labels are particularly appealing to health-conscious individuals, including those with chronic health issues like diabetes, as they promise a purer form of food without potentially harmful chemicals that might affect insulin sensitivity and overall health.

'Free-from' Claims

Labels stating a product is "free-from" indicate the absence of specific ingredients like gluten, dairy, or soy. For those with additional dietary restrictions apart from diabetes, these labels provide quick guidance. However, it's crucial to ensure that the removal of one ingredient hasn't led to the addition of another undesirable one—like sugar or artificial additives—that could sabotage your health goals.

Reading Between the Lines: Serving Sizes and Percent Daily Values

Serving sizes on food labels are not always representative of how much you might actually eat. It's important to adjust the nutritional information based on the actual portion you consume. Percent Daily Values (%DV) offer insight into how much a nutrient in a serving of food contributes to a daily diet. These percentages are based on a general 2,000-calorie per day diet, which might not necessarily apply to everyone, especially for those on a calorie-restricted diet for diabetes management.

Practical Application

To navigate the supermarket aisles armed with this information, consider implementing a few practical habits: - Always read the full label, not just the attractive claims on the front. - Compare products and choose ones with shorter ingredient lists and recognizable items. - Use a mobile app designed to scan barcodes and quickly display health information tailored to diabetes management.

Conclusion

The language of food labels is complex, but becoming fluent in it empowers you to make choices that profoundly impact your health and well-being. For those managing diabetes, these labels are not just lists of numbers and terms, but tools that enable informed decisions about food that support stable blood glucose levels and overall health. In essence, each label read correctly is a step towards a healthier life, ensuring that each meal nourishes and supports your body in the best ways possible.

REVITALIZING BREAKFAST RECIPES

Morning time can often feel like a rushed pause between waking and the full sprint of the day, especially when you're managing diabetes or prediabetes. Many think it's easier to skip breakfast, but let me be your guide to why revitalizing your morning meal can transform more than just your diet—it can change your entire approach to health and diabetic management.

Imagine the quiet of the morning; it's a blank slate. You have the opportunity to start your day in a way that supports your health and stabilizes

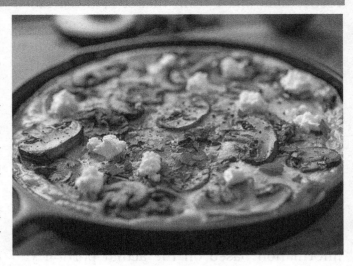

your blood sugar right from the beginning. Breakfast isn't just the first meal of the day; it's the foundational stone that can set the tone for your metabolic stability. Throughout this chapter, we'll explore ways to harness the power of breakfast so that it becomes a pleasure rather than a challenge.

We'll break down the essentials of a balanced diabetic-friendly breakfast, focusing on integrating proteins, fibers, and healthy fats that align with your low-carb, low-glycemic needs. But don't worry, this won't be a medical lecture! Instead, think of it as rediscovering the joy of morning meals through easy and quick recipes that are as delicious as they are nourishing.

Whether it's a speedy weekday smoothie enriched with greens and chia seeds, or a leisurely Sunday omelet stuffed with vibrant vegetables and sprinkled with herbs, the recipes you'll find here are designed to be both feasible and indulgent. I'll share some of my favorite quick fixes for those who don't want to spend their mornings in the kitchen, alongside some special weekend delights that you can savor with your family or friends.

Undoubtedly, the challenge of enjoying a breakfast that meets dietary restrictions can be daunting, but with a few tweaks and clever ideas, these recipes will not only satisfy your taste buds but also support your dietary goals, ensuring you start your day with a stable, satisfied feeling that carries you forward. Here's to mornings that energize and sustain us in more ways than one!

SAVORY MUSHROOM AND SPINACH FRITTATA

Preparation Time: 10 min
Cooking Time: 15 min
Servings: 2 Serv.
Glycemic Index: Low(~35)
Ingredients:

- 4 eggs
- 1 C. mushrooms, sliced
- 1 C. spinach, fresh
- 2 Tbsp onions, finely chopped
- 1 clove garlic, minced
- 2 Tbsp feta cheese, crumbled
- 1 Tbsp olive oil
- ½ tsp black pepper, ground

Directions:

1. Preheat oven to 375°F (190°C)
2. In a skillet, sauté onions, garlic, and mushrooms in olive oil until onions are translucent
3. Add spinach and cook until wilted
4. In a bowl, whisk eggs with black pepper, then pour over the vegetables in the skillet
5. Sprinkle crumbled feta on top
6. Transfer skillet to oven and bake for 15 min or until eggs are set

Tips:

- Garnish with fresh herbs for extra flavor
- Serve with a side of sliced avocado for additional healthy fats
- Remove from oven and let sit for a few minutes before serving to enhance flavors

Nutritional Values: Calories: 220, Fat: 16g, Carbs: 6g, Protein: 14g, Sugar: 2g, Sodium: 310mg, Potassium: 300mg, Cholesterol: 370mg

ALMOND AND COCONUT CHIA PUDDING

Preparation Time: 15 min
Cooking Time: none
Servings: 2
Glycemic Index: Low(~40)
Ingredients:

- 3 Tbsp chia seeds
- 1 C. unsweetened almond milk
- ¼ C. coconut flakes, unsweetened
- 1 tsp almond extract
- 1 Tbsp almond slivers, toasted
- 2 tsp erythritol

Directions:

1. Mix chia seeds, almond milk, coconut flakes, and almond extract in a bowl
2. Stir thoroughly to combine
3. Sweeten with erythritol and mix again
4. Cover and refrigerate overnight or at least for 4 hrs
5. Serve topped with toasted almond slivers

Tips:

- Experiment with different extracts like vanilla or hazelnut for variation in flavor
- Add fresh berries before serving for a fresh, fruity twist
- Stir every few hours while chilling to ensure evenly distributed chia seeds

Nutritional Values: Calories: 180, Fat: 12g, Carbs: 15g, Protein: 5g, Sugar: 1g, Sodium: 30mg, Potassium: 200mg, Cholesterol: 0mg

ZESTY TOMATO AND AVOCADO TOAST

Preparation Time: 5 min
Cooking Time: none
Servings: 2
Glycemic Index: Low(~55)
Ingredients:

- 2 slices whole grain bread
- 1 ripe avocado, mashed
- 1 tomato, sliced
- ½ tsp lemon zest
- 2 Tbsp crushed walnuts
- ½ tsp olive oil
- pinch of salt and black pepper

Directions:

1. Toast whole grain bread slices to desired crispness
2. Spread mashed avocado evenly on each slice
3. Layer with tomato slices
4. Drizzle with olive oil and sprinkle with lemon zest, salt, and black pepper
5. Garnish with crushed walnuts

Tips:

- Consider adding a sprinkle of chili flakes for a little heat
- Pair with a side of Greek yogurt for added protein
- Use ripe, flavorful tomatoes for the best taste

Nutritional Values: Calories: 250, Fat: 15g, Carbs: 27g, Protein: 6g, Sugar: 4g, Sodium: 200mg, Potassium: 500mg, Cholesterol: 0mg

HERBED TURKEY AND SPINACH MINI QUICHES

Preparation Time: 15 min
Cooking Time: 20 min
Servings: 4
Glycemic Index: Low(~30)
Ingredients:

- 4 eggs
- ½ C. milk, skimmed
- 1 C. turkey, cooked and chopped
- 1 C. spinach, fresh
- 1 Tbsp chives, chopped
- 1 Tbsp parsley, chopped
- ¼ tsp nutmeg
- 1/2 cup diced bell peppers
- salt and pepper to taste

Directions:

1. Preheat oven to 350°F (175°C)
2. Whisk eggs and milk together in a bowl
3. Stir in chopped turkey, spinach, chives, parsley, bell peppers, nutmeg, salt, and pepper
4. Pour mixture into greased mini muffin tins
5. Bake for 20 min or until set

Tips:

- Serve warm or store in the refrigerator for a quick grab-and-go option
- Enhance flavor with a sprinkle of grated Parmesan before baking if desired
- Pair with a mixed greens salad for a complete meal

Nutritional Values: Calories: 110, Fat: 5g, Carbs: 3g, Protein: 13g, Sugar: 2g, Sodium: 125mg, Potassium: 180mg, Cholesterol: 184mg

CHIA AND COCONUT YOGURT PARFAIT

Preparation Time: 10 min
Cooking Time: none
Servings: 2
Glycemic Index: Low(~35)
Ingredients:

- 1 C. Greek yogurt, unsweetened
- 3 Tbsp chia seeds
- ½ C. coconut flakes, unsweetened
- ¼ C. almonds, chopped
- 1 tsp vanilla extract
- 2 Tbsp shredded coconut for topping
- 1 C. mixed berries (blueberries, raspberries)

Directions:

1. Mix Greek yogurt with chia seeds, vanilla extract, and half of the coconut flakes in a bowl until well combined
2. Let sit for about 5 minutes to allow chia seeds to swell
3. Layer the yogurt mixture in two glasses alternating with mixed berries and remaining coconut flakes
4. Top with chopped almonds and shredded coconut
5. Serve chilled

Tips:

- Add a pinch of cinnamon to the yogurt mixture for extra flavor
- Consider using a mix of seeds like flax or pumpkin for varied texture and increased nutritional benefits

Nutritional Values: Calories: 310, Fat: 19g, Carbs: 23g, Protein: 13g, Sugar: 8g, Sodium: 45mg, Potassium: 350mg, Cholesterol: 10mg

SAVORY SPINACH AND MUSHROOM EGG MUFFINS

Preparation Time: 15 min
Cooking Time: 20 min
Servings: 6
Glycemic Index: Low(~50)
Ingredients:

- 6 eggs
- 1 C. spinach, chopped
- ½ C. mushrooms, diced
- ⅓ C. feta cheese, crumbled
- ¼ C. red bell pepper, diced
- Salt and pepper to taste
- Olive oil spray for muffin tin

Directions:

1. Preheat oven to 375°F (190°C)
2. Whisk eggs in a large bowl and season with salt and pepper
3. Add spinach, mushrooms, feta cheese, and red bell pepper to the egg mixture and stir to combine
4. Lightly spray a 6-cup muffin tin with olive oil and evenly distribute the egg mixture among the cups
5. Bake for 20 minutes or until the muffins are set and lightly golden on top
6. Let them cool in pan for 5 minutes before serving

Tips:

- Serve with a side of fresh salsa for added zest
- Store leftovers in the refrigerator for a quick breakfast option on busy mornings

Nutritional Values: Calories: 140, Fat: 9g, Carbs: 3g, Protein: 12g, Sugar: 2g, Sodium: 200mg, Potassium: 180mg, Cholesterol: 215mg

CINNAMON ALMOND FLAX PANCAKES

Preparation Time: 15 min
Cooking Time: 10 min
Servings: 4
Glycemic Index: Low(~45)
Ingredients:

- ¾ C. almond flour
- ¼ C. flaxseed meal
- 2 eggs
- ½ C. unsweetened almond milk
- 1 tsp cinnamon, ground
- 1 Tbsp erythritol
- 2 tsp baking powder
- Olive oil spray for cooking

Directions:

1. Combine almond flour, flaxseed meal, baking powder, cinnamon, and erythritol in a bowl
2. In another bowl, whisk eggs and almond milk together
3. Mix dry and wet ingredients until a smooth batter forms
4. Heat a non-stick skillet over medium heat and spray with olive oil
5. Pour ¼ C. of batter for each pancake and cook for about 2-3 minutes per side or until golden and fluffy
6. Serve hot

Tips:

- Consider adding a small amount of nutmeg or vanilla extract to the batter for enhanced flavor
- Serve with a dollop of low-carb Greek yogurt and a sprinkle of nuts

Nutritional Values: Calories: 220, Fat: 18g, Carbs: 8g, Protein: 10g, Sugar: 1g, Sodium: 60mg, Potassium: 300mg, Cholesterol: 95mg

ZUCCHINI AND HERB BREAKFAST HASH

Preparation Time: 10 min
Cooking Time: 15 min
Servings: 4
Glycemic Index: Low(~55)
Ingredients:

- 2 C. zucchini, cubed
- 1 C. bell peppers, mixed colors, diced
- 1 medium onion, diced
- 2 garlic cloves, minced
- 4 eggs
- 2 Tbsp olive oil
- 1 tsp thyme, dried
- Salt and pepper to taste

Directions:

1. Heat olive oil in a large skillet over medium heat
2. Add onion and garlic, sauté until translucent
3. Increase heat to medium-high, add zucchini and bell peppers, cook until slightly browned and tender, stirring occasionally
4. Create four wells in the hash, crack an egg into each, cover the skillet and cook until eggs are set to your liking
5. Season with thyme, salt, and pepper
6. Serve hot

Tips:

- Customize with additional herbs like rosemary or oregano for different flavors
- Serve alongside whole-grain toast for added fiber if not strictly low-carb

Nutritional Values: Calories: 220, Fat: 15g, Carbs: 10g, Protein: 11g, Sugar: 6g, Sodium: 125mg, Potassium: 450mg, Cholesterol: 190mg

ZUCCHINI AND BELL PEPPER MINI FRITTATAS

Preparation Time: 10 min
Cooking Time: 20 min
Servings: 6
Glycemic Index: Low(~35)
Ingredients:

- 6 eggs, whisked
- 1 C. zucchini, grated
- 1 C. bell pepper, diced
- ¼ C. feta cheese, crumbled
- 2 Tbsp fresh parsley, chopped
- 1 tsp olive oil
- ¼ tsp black pepper
- ⅛ tsp salt

Directions:

1. Preheat oven to 375°F (190°C)
2. Grease a 12-cup muffin pan with olive oil
3. Mix eggs, zucchini, bell pepper, feta cheese, parsley, black pepper, and salt in a bowl
4. Pour the mixture into the muffin cups, filling each about two-thirds full
5. Bake for 20 min or until the eggs are set and the tops are slightly golden

Tips:

- Add a pinch of paprika for a bit of warmth and color
- Consider substituting zucchini with shredded carrot for a sweeter taste
- Serve with a side of mixed greens for a complete meal

Nutritional Values: Calories: 100, Fat: 7g, Carbs: 3g, Protein: 6g, Sugar: 2g, Sodium: 150mg, Potassium: 200mg, Cholesterol: 170mg

CHIA AND BERRY YOGURT PARFAIT

Preparation Time: 10 min
Cooking Time: none
Servings: 1
Glycemic Index: Low(~35)
Ingredients:

- ¾ C. Greek yogurt, unsweetened
- 2 Tbsp chia seeds
- ½ C. mixed berries (blueberries, raspberries)
- 1 Tbsp sliced almonds
- 1 tsp vanilla extract
- 1 Tbsp coconut flakes, unsweetened

Directions:

1. Mix Greek yogurt with vanilla extract and chia seeds in a bowl until well combined
2. In a serving glass, layer half of the yogurt mixture
3. Add a layer of mixed berries
4. Repeat with the remaining yogurt and top with the remaining berries
5. Sprinkle sliced almonds and coconut flakes on top
6. Serve immediately or chill in the refrigerator for 15 minutes if preferred

Tips:

- To enhance the sweetness naturally, allow the parfait to rest for a few minutes after assembly to let the berries release their natural juices
- For a nut-free option, substitute almonds with pumpkin seeds
- Increase the fiber content by adding a layer of flaxseed meal between the yogurt layers

Nutritional Values: Calories: 290, Fat: 15g, Carbs: 25g, Protein: 18g, Sugar: 12g, Sodium: 85mg, Potassium: 345mg, Cholesterol: 10mg

SPINACH AND FETA BREAKFAST WRAP

Preparation Time: 15 min
Cooking Time: 5 min
Servings: 1
Glycemic Index: Medium(~65)
Ingredients:

- 1 large whole wheat tortilla
- 1 C. spinach, fresh
- ¼ C. feta cheese, crumbled
- 2 egg whites
- 1 Tbsp olive oil
- 1 tsp lemon zest
- Salt and pepper to taste

Directions:

1. Heat olive oil in a skillet over medium heat
2. Add spinach and cook until just wilted, about 2 min
3. In a separate bowl, whisk egg whites with lemon zest, salt, and pepper
4. Add egg mixture to skillet and scramble together with spinach until eggs are set, about 3 min
5. Warm tortilla in microwave for 10 sec
6. Place the spinach and egg mixture on the tortilla, sprinkle feta cheese on top
7. Roll up the tortilla tightly and serve warm

Tips:

- Wrap can be prepared the night before and quickly warmed in the morning for an even faster breakfast
- Add diced tomatoes for a fresh, juicy touch
- Sprinkle some chili flakes for an extra kick if you enjoy a bit of spice

Nutritional Values: Calories: 330, Fat: 18g, Carbs: 24g, Protein: 20g, Sugar: 3g, Sodium: 580mg, Potassium: 465mg, Cholesterol: 25mg

ALMOND BUTTER AND BANANA OPEN SANDWICH

Preparation Time: 5 min
Cooking Time: none
Servings: 1
Glycemic Index: Medium(~61)
Ingredients:

- 1 slice of whole grain bread, toasted
- 2 Tbsp almond butter
- 1 small banana, sliced
- 1 tsp chia seeds
- 1 Tbsp honey, optional (considered for GI calculations)

Directions:

1. Spread almond butter evenly over the toasted whole grain bread
2. Arrange sliced banana on top of the almond butter
3. Sprinkle chia seeds over the banana slices
4. Drizzle honey over the top if using, though considering the diabetic-friendly focus, the honey can be omitted or replaced with a drizzle of a low-GI sweetener like monk fruit extract

Tips:

- To boost protein, add a sprinkle of hemp seeds along with the chia seeds
- For more texture, include a few crushed walnuts on top
- Remember, if using honey, use sparingly and be mindful of portion size to maintain lower GI

Nutritional Values: Calories: 345, Fat: 18g, Carbs: 37g, Protein: 8g, Sugar: 19g (less if omitting or substituting honey), Sodium: 150mg, Potassium: 422mg, Cholesterol: 0mg

Savory Cottage Cheese Bowl

Preparation Time: 10 min
Cooking Time: none
Servings: 1
Glycemic Index: Low(~45)
Ingredients:

- ½ C. cottage cheese, low-fat
- ¼ C. cherry tomatoes, halved
- 2 Tbsp avocado, diced
- 1 Tbsp green onions, chopped
- Salt and pepper to taste
- 1 tsp olive oil

Directions:

1. In a bowl, combine cottage cheese with salt, pepper, and olive oil
2. Gently fold in cherry tomatoes, avocado, and green onions until well mixed
3. Serve chilled or at room temperature as a refreshing and filling start to your day

Tips:

- Experiment with other vegetables like diced cucumbers or shredded carrots for different flavors and textures
- A sprinkle of paprika or dried basil can add an interesting twist to the dish
- If more texture is desired, add a tablespoon of roasted sunflower seeds

Nutritional Values: Calories: 190, Fat: 10g, Carbs: 9g, Protein: 14g, Sugar: 5g, Sodium: 390mg, Potassium: 200mg, Cholesterol: 5mg

Almond Flour Pancakes with Berry Compote

Preparation Time: 15 min
Cooking Time: 10 min
Servings: 2
Glycemic Index: Low(~45)
Ingredients:

- ¾ C. almond flour
- 2 eggs
- ¼ C. water
- 1 tsp baking powder
- 1 Tbsp olive oil
- 1 C. fresh strawberries, hulled and sliced
- 1 Tbsp erythritol
- Juice of half a lemon

Directions:

1. In a bowl, mix almond flour, eggs, water, baking powder until smooth for the pancake batter
2. Heat olive oil in a skillet over medium heat and pour in batter to form pancakes, cook until golden on both sides, approximately 2-3 min per side
3. For the compote, combine strawberries, erythritol, and lemon juice in a saucepan over medium heat, stir until berries break down and the mixture thickens, about 8 min
4. Serve pancakes topped with the berry compote

Tips:

- Use blueberries or raspberries for variety in the compote
- For fluffier pancakes, separate the eggs, whisk the whites, and fold them into the batter
- Serve with a dollop of diabetic-friendly whipped cream for added indulgence

Nutritional Values: Calories: 320, Fat: 25g, Carbs: 18g, Protein: 12g, Sugar: 5g, Sodium: 300mg, Potassium: 150mg, Cholesterol: 122mg

SAVORY SPINACH AND FETA MUFFINS

Preparation Time: 15 min
Cooking Time: 25 min
Servings: 4
Glycemic Index: Low(~40)
Ingredients:

- 1½ C. almond flour
- 3 eggs
- ½ C. spinach, chopped
- ¼ C. feta cheese, crumbled
- 1 Tbsp olive oil
- 1 tsp baking powder
- 1 small onion, finely chopped
- Salt and pepper to taste
- Non-stick cooking spray

Directions:

1. Preheat oven to 375°F (190°C)
2. Saute onion in olive oil until translucent, about 5 min, and set aside to cool
3. In a bowl, whisk eggs and then mix in almond flour, baking powder, cooled onion, spinach, feta, salt, and pepper
4. Spray a muffin tin with non-stick spray and divide mixture among cups
5. Bake for 20-25 min until tops are golden and a tester comes out clean
6. Serve warm

Tips:

- Experiment with different herbs like dill or chives for added flavor
- These muffins can be frozen and reheated for a quick breakfast option
- Adding chopped sun-dried tomatoes can enhance flavor and texture

Nutritional Values: Calories: 200, Fat: 15g, Carbs: 10g, Protein: 9g, Sugar: 2g, Sodium: 220mg, Potassium: 50mg, Cholesterol: 170mg

SMOKED SALMON AND AVOCADO WRAP

Preparation Time: 10 min
Cooking Time: none
Servings: 1
Glycemic Index: Low(~40)
Ingredients:

- 1 low-carb whole wheat wrap
- 3 oz. smoked salmon
- ½ avocado, sliced
- ½ C. arugula
- 1 Tbsp cream cheese, low-fat
- 1 tsp lemon juice
- Salt and pepper to taste

Directions:

1. Spread cream cheese over the surface of the wrap
2. Lay down slices of avocado on top of the cream cheese
3. Add smoked salmon and arugula, sprinkle with lemon juice, salt, and pepper
4. Roll the wrap tightly and slice into halves before serving

Tips:

- For a zestier flavor, add a few capers or a sprinkle of red onion
- Use spinach instead of arugula for a milder taste
- A drizzle of olive oil can be used instead of lemon juice for extra richness

Nutritional Values: Calories: 290, Fat: 17g, Carbs: 20g, Protein: 18g, Sugar: 2g, Sodium: 710mg, Potassium: 500mg, Cholesterol: 30mg

SPINACH AND FETA BREAKFAST WRAPS

Preparation Time: 15 min
Cooking Time: 5 min
Servings: 2
Glycemic Index: Low(~30)
Ingredients:

- 2 whole wheat tortillas
- 1 cup spinach, fresh
- ½ cup feta cheese, crumbled
- 4 egg whites
- 1 Tbsp olive oil
- 1 small onion, finely chopped
- Salt and pepper to taste

Directions:

1. Heat olive oil in a non-stick pan over medium heat
2. Sauté onions until translucent
3. Add spinach and cook until wilted
4. Whisk egg whites and pour over the spinach, stirring until the eggs are fully cooked
5. Season with salt and pepper
6. Divide the scramble between the tortillas, sprinkle feta cheese on top, and fold into wraps

Tips:

- Cook extra portions and store in the fridge for a quick reheat during busy mornings
- Personalize with different veggies like bell peppers or zucchini for extra nutrition
- Add a dash of hot sauce for a spicy kick

Nutritional Values: Calories: 290, Fat: 15g, Carbs: 20g, Protein: 18g, Sugar: 3g, Sodium: 620mg, Potassium: 300mg, Cholesterol: 10mg

ALMOND BUTTER AND BANANA TOAST

Preparation Time: 5 min
Cooking Time: 2 min
Servings: 1
Glycemic Index: Low(~40)
Ingredients:

- 1 slice of whole grain bread
- 2 Tbsp almond butter, smooth
- 1 banana, sliced
- 1 tsp honey, optional
- Sprinkle of flaxseeds

Directions:

1. Toast whole grain bread to desired crispiness
2. Spread almond butter evenly over the toasted slice
3. Arrange banana slices on top of the almond butter
4. Drizzle with honey if using, and sprinkle flaxseeds for added texture and nutrients

Tips:

- Substitute honey with a drizzle of agave if preferred for a slightly lower GI option
- Press banana slices slightly into the almond butter to prevent them from sliding off while eating
- Pair this toast with a cup of unsweetened herbal tea for a complete breakfast

Nutritional Values: Calories: 280, Fat: 14g, Carbs: 32g, Protein: 8g, Sugar: 10g, Sodium: 180mg, Potassium: 400mg, Cholesterol: 0mg

ZUCCHINI AND GOAT CHEESE FRITTATA

Preparation Time: 15 min
Cooking Time: 15 min
Servings: 2
Glycemic Index: Low(~45)
Ingredients:

- 4 eggs, whisked
- 1 medium zucchini, thinly sliced
- 2 oz. goat cheese, crumbled
- 1 small onion, diced
- 1 clove garlic, minced
- 2 tsp olive oil
- 1/4 tsp salt
- 1/4 tsp black pepper

Directions:

1. Preheat oven to 375°F (190°C)
2. Heat olive oil in a 10-inch ovenproof skillet over medium heat
3. Add onion and garlic, sauté until translucent
4. Add zucchini slices and cook until tender
5. Pour whisked eggs over vegetables in skillet
6. Crumble goat cheese on top
7. Season with salt and pepper
8. Transfer skillet to oven and bake until frittata is set, about 15 min
9. Remove from oven, let cool slightly before slicing and serving

Tips:

- Consider adding a pinch of nutmeg or smoked paprika for an intriguing flavor twist
- Serve with a side of mixed greens for a complete meal
- Leftovers make a great quick breakfast or lunch option

Nutritional Values: Calories: 310, Fat: 20g, Carbs: 8g, Protein: 23g, Sugar: 4g, Sodium: 430mg, Potassium: 300mg, Cholesterol: 370mg

ALMOND FLOUR BLUEBERRY PANCAKES

Preparation Time: 10 min
Cooking Time: 15 min
Servings: 2
Glycemic Index: Low(~35)
Ingredients:

- 1 cup almond flour
- 2 eggs
- 1/3 cup almond milk, unsweetened
- 1/2 cup blueberries, fresh
- 1 tsp vanilla extract
- 1 tsp baking powder
- 1 Tbsp erythritol
- 2 tsp coconut oil

Directions:

1. In a bowl, mix almond flour, eggs, almond milk, vanilla extract, baking powder, and erythritol until smooth
2. Heat a skillet over medium heat and add coconut oil
3. Pour batter to form small pancakes, about 1/4 cup each
4. Drop blueberries onto each pancake
5. Cook until bubbles form on top, about 3 min per side, then flip and cook until golden brown

Tips:

- Use fresh or frozen blueberries but ensure they are not added frozen to the batter to prevent sogginess
- If the batter is too thick, add a bit more almond milk for a desired consistency
- Serve with a dollop of Greek yogurt for extra protein

Nutritional Values: Calories: 250, Fat: 18g, Carbs: 16g, Protein: 12g, Sugar: 2g, Sodium: 150mg, Potassium: 100mg, Cholesterol: 180mg

SHAKSHUKA WITH SPINACH AND FETA

Preparation Time: 10 min
Cooking Time: 20 min
Servings: 2
Glycemic Index: Low(~38)
Ingredients:

- 4 eggs
- 1 can (14 oz.) diced tomatoes
- 2 cups spinach, chopped
- 1/2 cup feta cheese, crumbled
- 1 small onion, chopped
- 2 cloves garlic, minced
- 2 tsp olive oil
- 1 tsp smoked paprika
- 1 tsp cumin
- Salt and pepper to taste

Directions:

1. Heat olive oil in a deep skillet over medium heat
2. Add onion and garlic, cook until softened
3. Stir in smoked paprika and cumin, cook for 1 min
4. Add diced tomatoes and bring to a simmer
5. Stir in spinach until wilted
6. Make four wells in the sauce and crack an egg into each
7. Sprinkle crumbled feta around the eggs
8. Cover and simmer until eggs are set, about 10 min
9. Season with salt and pepper to taste

Tips:

- Add a sprinkle of chili flakes for a spicy kick
- Serve with low-GI toast or a side salad
- Can be stored in the refrigerator and reheated for up to two days

Nutritional Values: Calories: 290, Fat: 18g, Carbs: 12g, Protein: 19g, Sugar: 5g, Sodium: 610mg, Potassium: 500mg, Cholesterol: 370mg

COCONUT YOGURT PARFAIT WITH KIWI AND WALNUTS

Preparation Time: 5 min
Cooking Time: none
Servings: 1
Glycemic Index: Low(~39)
Ingredients:

- 1 cup coconut yogurt, unsweetened
- 1 kiwi, peeled and sliced
- 1/4 cup walnuts, chopped
- 1 tsp chia seeds
- 1 Tbsp coconut flakes, unsweetened

Directions:

1. In a glass, layer half of the coconut yogurt at the bottom
2. Add a layer of sliced kiwi and a sprinkle of chopped walnuts
3. Add another layer of yogurt and repeat the kiwi and walnut layers
4. Top with chia seeds and coconut flakes

Tips:

- Experiment with different fruits like berries or pomegranate for variety
- Keep ingredients separate until ready to eat to maintain freshness
- Try toasting the walnuts for added crunch and deeper flavor

Nutritional Values: Calories: 360, Fat: 26g, Carbs: 24g, Protein: 8g, Sugar: 13g, Sodium: 30mg, Potassium: 500mg, Cholesterol: 0mg

RICOTTA AND CHIVE CLOUD PANCAKES

Preparation Time: 15 min
Cooking Time: 10 min
Servings: 2
Glycemic Index: Low(~45)
Ingredients:

- 1 C. ricotta cheese
- 2 large eggs, separated
- 1/4 C. almond flour
- 1 tsp baking powder
- 2 Tbsp chives, finely chopped
- 1/4 tsp salt
- 1/2 tsp lemon zest
- Olive oil for cooking

Directions:

1. Whisk egg yolks with ricotta cheese until smooth
2. Mix almond flour, baking powder, salt, chives, and lemon zest in a separate bowl
3. Combine both mixtures gently
4. In another bowl, beat egg whites to stiff peaks
5. Fold egg whites into the batter for airiness
6. Heat a nonstick skillet and brush with olive oil
7. Pour batter to form small pancakes, cooking until golden on both sides and fluffy
8. Serve warm with a dollop of unsweetened Greek yogurt or drizzle of low-carb syrup

Tips:

- Experiment with different herbs like dill or parsley for a new flavor profile
- Serve alongside mixed berries for added freshness and a slight natural sweetness
- Ensure not to over-mix the batter after adding egg whites to keep pancakes light and airy

Nutritional Values: Calories: 310, Fat: 22g, Carbs: 8g, Protein: 18g, Sugar: 2g, Sodium: 410mg, Potassium: 200mg, Cholesterol: 190mg

MUSHROOM AND SPINACH FRITTATA

Preparation Time: 10 min
Cooking Time: 20 min
Servings: 4
Glycemic Index: Low(~40)
Ingredients:

- 6 large eggs
- 1 C. mushrooms, sliced
- 1 C. spinach, fresh
- 1/2 C. feta cheese, crumbled
- 1/4 C. milk, almond or soy
- 1 tsp garlic, minced
- 2 Tbsp olive oil
- Salt and pepper to taste

Directions:

1. Preheat oven to 375°F (190°C)
2. Sauté mushrooms and garlic in olive oil until tender
3. Add spinach and cook until wilted
4. Beat eggs with milk, salt, and pepper
5. Pour eggs over vegetables in a non-stick baking dish
6. Sprinkle feta cheese on top
7. Bake for 20 min or until the eggs are set and top is lightly browned

Tips:

- Add a sprinkle of crushed red pepper flakes for a spicy kick
- Pair with a side of avocado slices for healthy fats
- Can be made in advance and reheated for a quick and nutritious breakfast

Nutritional Values: Calories: 230, Fat: 17g, Carbs: 6g, Protein: 14g, Sugar: 3g, Sodium: 420mg, Potassium: 300mg, Cholesterol: 370mg

ALMOND AND COCONUT FLOUR WAFFLES

Preparation Time: 10 min
Cooking Time: 15 min
Servings: 3
Glycemic Index: Low(~45)
Ingredients:

- 1/2 C. almond flour
- 1/2 C. coconut flour
- 2 large eggs
- 1/3 C. unsweetened almond milk
- 1 tsp vanilla extract
- 1 Tbsp erythritol
- 2 tsp baking powder
- 1/4 C. unsalted butter, melted
- Dash of salt

Directions:

1. Mix almond flour, coconut flour, baking powder, and salt in a bowl
2. In another bowl, whisk eggs, almond milk, melted butter, erythritol, and vanilla extract
3. Combine wet and dry ingredients until smooth
4. Heat waffle iron and lightly grease it
5. Pour batter and cook each waffle until golden brown and crisp

Tips:

- Serve with a dollop of sugar-free whipped cream
- Add cinnamon or nutmeg to the batter for extra flavor
- Keep waffles warm in the oven at a low temperature while finishing the batch to serve them all hot at once

Nutritional Values: Calories: 280, Fat: 22g, Carbs: 15g, Protein: 9g, Sugar: 2g, Sodium: 300mg, Potassium: 100mg, Cholesterol: 185mg

SAVORY YOGURT BOWL WITH ROASTED VEGGIES

Preparation Time: 20 min
Cooking Time: none
Servings: 1
Glycemic Index: Low(~35)
Ingredients:

- 1 C. Greek yogurt, unsweetened
- 1/2 C. roasted vegetables (red peppers, zucchini, onions)
- 2 Tbsp pumpkin seeds
- 1 Tbsp olive oil
- 1/2 tsp smoked paprika
- Salt and pepper to taste
- Fresh herbs for garnish (such as parsley or cilantro)

Directions:

1. Toss roasted vegetables with olive oil, smoked paprika, salt, and pepper
2. Place Greek yogurt in a bowl
3. Top with seasoned roasted vegetables
4. Sprinkle pumpkin seeds and fresh herbs on top
5. Drizzle with a little more olive oil if desired

Tips:

- Personalize with different vegetables such as broccoli or cherry tomatoes depending on seasonal availability
- Add a sprinkle of feta or goat cheese for a creamy texture and tangy flavor
- Try using different nuts or seeds like walnuts or sunflower seeds for variety

Nutritional Values: Calories: 290, Fat: 19g, Carbs: 13g, Protein: 17g, Sugar: 6g, Sodium: 170mg, Potassium: 350mg, Cholesterol: 10mg

ZUCCHINI RICOTTA PANCAKES

Preparation Time: 15 min
Cooking Time: 10 min
Servings: 4
Glycemic Index: Low(~30)
Ingredients:

- 2 medium zucchini, grated
- 1 cup whole-milk ricotta
- 2 eggs, beaten
- 4 Tbsp almond flour
- 1 tsp garlic powder
- 1/4 tsp salt
- 1/4 tsp black pepper
- 2 Tbsp olive oil for cooking

Directions:

1. Grate zucchini and squeeze out extra moisture with a clean cloth
2. In a mixing bowl, combine grated zucchini, ricotta, beaten eggs, almond flour, garlic powder, salt, and pepper, and stir until well mixed
3. Heat olive oil in a skillet over medium heat
4. Scoop 1/4 cup of batter for each pancake into the skillet and flatten lightly with the back of a spatula
5. Cook for about 5 min on each side or until golden brown and cooked through
6. Serve warm

Tips:

- Add a dollop of unsweetened Greek yogurt on top for extra creaminess
- Sprinkle fresh chives or parsley for a touch of freshness
- These pancakes can be made in advance and reheated for a quick breakfast

Nutritional Values: Calories: 220, Fat: 17g, Carbs: 7g, Protein: 11g, Sugar: 4g, Sodium: 320mg, Potassium: 340mg, Cholesterol: 90mg

LUNCH RECIPES THAT NOURISH AND SATISFY

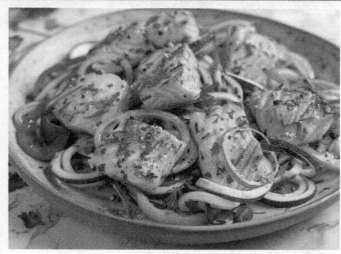

When the midday hunger pangs strike, there's a real temptation to grab whatever is quickest — often leading us down a path lined with unhealthy choices. However, lunch represents a pivotal opportunity to nourish your body and maintain your energy levels throughout the day, especially important for those managing diabetes or prediabetes. Imagine a lunch that satisfies not just your taste buds but also stabilizes your blood sugar and keeps you fueled till dinner. That's what this chapter aims to provide: delicious, diabetic-friendly lunch recipes that are both nutritious and heartwarming.

In our golden years, lunch takes on new significance. As metabolism naturally changes, each meal's impact on our blood sugar becomes more pronounced. Therefore, selecting the right ingredients and preparing meals that blend taste with nutritional value is more crucial than ever. This is not just about avoiding spikes in your glucose levels; it's about enjoying vibrant plates of food that look as good as they taste—meals that you can share with family and friends without them even realizing they are "diabetic-friendly."

From hearty, warm soups that hug your soul to crisp, fresh salads that burst with color and flavor, these recipes are designed to keep you satisfied without the post-lunch slump. We'll explore how traditional dishes can be adapted to fit a low-carb, low-glycemic profile while still retaining all the flavors and textures you love. For instance, imagine a creamy mushroom soup that uses aromatic herbs and spices to compensate for less cream or a zesty chicken salad dressed in a light, tangy vinaigrette instead of a heavy, sugary dressing.

But it's not just about the dishes themselves—it's the stories they tell and the smiles they bring. Each recipe in this section is more than a set of instructions; it's a passport to a healthier, more joyful way of eating. So, let's embrace this lunchtime journey together. Prepare your taste buds for delight and your body for nourishment—the kind that only well-crafted, mindful eating can provide.

CHILLED ZUCCHINI NOODLE SALAD WITH FLAKED SALMON

Preparation Time: 15 min
Cooking Time: none
Servings: 2
Glycemic Index: Low(~35)
Ingredients:

- 2 large zucchini, spiralized
- 6 oz. salmon, cooked and flaked
- 1 red bell pepper, thinly sliced
- 1/4 cup red onion, finely chopped
- 2 Tbsp extra virgin olive oil
- 2 Tbsp apple cider vinegar
- 1 tsp Dijon mustard
- Salt and pepper to taste

Directions:

1. Spiralize zucchinis and set aside in a large mixing bowl
2. Add the thinly sliced red bell pepper and chopped red onion to the zucchini noodles
3. In a small bowl, whisk together extra virgin olive oil, apple cider vinegar, and Dijon mustard until emulsified
4. Pour dressing over zucchini noodles and toss to coat evenly
5. Gently mix in flaked salmon and season with salt and pepper
6. Chill in the refrigerator for about 10 minutes before serving to enhance flavors

Tips:

- Opt for wild-caught salmon for higher omega-3 content
- Add a sprinkle of chopped fresh herbs like dill or parsley before serving for extra flavor
- Use a vegetable peeler if you don't have a spiralizer to create thin zucchini ribbons

Nutritional Values: Calories: 310, Fat: 18g, Carbs: 12g, Protein: 22g, Sugar: 6g, Sodium: 80mg, Potassium: 800mg, Cholesterol: 40mg

HEARTY TURKEY AND WHITE BEAN CHILI

Preparation Time: 10 min
Cooking Time: 20 min
Servings: 4
Glycemic Index: Low(~55)
Ingredients:

- 1 lb ground turkey
- 1 onion, diced
- 2 cloves garlic, minced
- 1 can (15 oz.) white beans, drained and rinsed
- 1 can (14.5 oz.) diced tomatoes with juice
- 1 Tbsp chili powder
- 1 tsp ground cumin
- 2 cups low-sodium chicken broth
- Salt and pepper to taste

Directions:

1. In a large pot, sauté ground turkey, diced onion, and minced garlic over medium heat until turkey is browned and onions are translucent
2. Stir in chili powder and ground cumin, cooking for another 1 min
3. Add white beans, diced tomatoes with their juice, and low-sodium chicken broth
4. Bring chili to a simmer and let cook for 20 min, stirring occasionally
5. Season with salt and pepper to taste and serve hot

Tips:

- To thicken the chili, mash some of the white beans before adding them to the pot
- Serve with a slice of whole-grain bread for additional fiber
- Garnish with a dollop of low-fat Greek yogurt for extra creaminess

Nutritional Values: Calories: 350, Fat: 8g, Carbs: 30g, Protein: 35g, Sugar: 4g, Sodium: 400mg, Potassium: 950mg, Cholesterol: 60mg

ASIAN SHRIMP AND SNOW PEA STIR-FRY

Preparation Time: 10 min
Cooking Time: 10 min
Servings: 3
Glycemic Index: Low(~45)
Ingredients:

- 12 oz. shelled and deveined shrimp
- 2 cups snow peas, trimmed
- 1 bell pepper, julienned
- 1 Tbsp ginger, freshly grated
- 2 Tbsp low-sodium soy sauce
- 1 Tbsp sesame oil
- 1 tsp sesame seeds
- 1/4 cup scallions, chopped

Directions:

1. Heat sesame oil in a wok or large frying pan over medium-high heat
2. Add freshly grated ginger and julienned bell pepper, stir-fry for 2 min
3. Add shrimp and stir-fry until they turn pink, about 3-4 min
4. Add snow peas and continue to stir-fry for another 3 min
5. Pour low-sodium soy sauce over the mixture, stir well to coat
6. Sprinkle sesame seeds and chopped scallions before serving

Tips:

- Ensure shrimp are patted dry to avoid steaming instead of stir-frying
- Substitute shrimp with tofu for a vegetarian option
- Add a splash of lime juice for a zesty flavor boost

Nutritional Values: Calories: 200, Fat: 8g, Carbs: 10g, Protein: 20g, Sugar: 5g, Sodium: 300mg, Potassium: 400mg, Cholesterol: 120mg

SPICED LENTIL SOUP WITH SPINACH

Preparation Time: 15 min
Cooking Time: 15 min
Servings: 4
Glycemic Index: Low(~30)
Ingredients:

- 2 cups lentils, rinsed
- 4 cups vegetable broth
- 1 cup spinach, chopped
- 1 carrot, diced
- 1 onion, chopped
- 2 cloves garlic, minced
- 1 tsp turmeric
- 1 tsp ground coriander
- 1/2 tsp cayenne pepper
- Salt and pepper to taste

Directions:

1. Place rinsed lentils in a large pot with vegetable broth and bring to a boil over high heat
2. Reduce heat to medium-low and add diced carrot, chopped onion, and minced garlic to the pot, simmer for 10 min until lentils are tender
3. Stir in turmeric, ground coriander, and cayenne pepper
4. Add chopped spinach and cook for another 5 min
5. Season with salt and pepper to taste and serve hot

Tips:

- Use a pressure cooker to reduce cooking time significantly
- Blend half of the soup before adding spinach for a creamier texture
- Add a squeeze of lemon juice before serving to enhance flavors

Nutritional Values: Calories: 250, Fat: 2g, Carbs: 40g, Protein: 18g, Sugar: 3g, Sodium: 300mg, Potassium: 700mg, Cholesterol: 0mg

CHILLED AVOCADO SOUP WITH LIME AND CILANTRO

Preparation Time: 10 min
Cooking Time: none
Servings: 4
Glycemic Index: Low(~40)
Ingredients:

- 2 avocados, ripe and pitted
- 1 C. cucumber, peeled and chopped
- 1 garlic clove, minced
- 2 cups plain yogurt, low-fat
- Juice of 2 limes
- ½ C. cilantro, chopped
- 1 tsp cumin, ground
- 1 C. vegetable broth, low sodium
- Salt and pepper to taste

Directions:

1. Combine avocados, cucumber, garlic, yogurt, lime juice, cilantro, cumin, and vegetable broth in a blender
2. Blend until smooth
3. Season with salt and pepper to taste
4. Chill in the refrigerator for at least 30 minutes before serving

Tips:

- Serve chilled for a refreshing lunch option
- Garnish with extra cilantro or a slice of lime for an elegant touch
- For a creamier texture, add more yogurt

Nutritional Values: Calories: 190, Fat: 12g, Carbs: 15g, Protein: 6g, Sugar: 6g, Sodium: 150mg, Potassium: 450mg, Cholesterol: 10mg

MEDITERRANEAN CHICKPEA SALAD

Preparation Time: 15 min
Cooking Time: none
Servings: 4
Glycemic Index: Low(~55)
Ingredients:

- 1 can chickpeas, drained and rinsed
- 1 red bell pepper, diced
- 1 C. cherry tomatoes, halved
- ½ red onion, thinly sliced
- ¼ C. black olives, pitted and sliced
- 2 Tbsp olive oil
- 1 Tbsp red wine vinegar
- 1 clove garlic, minced
- 1 tsp dried oregano
- Salt and pepper to taste

Directions:

1. Combine chickpeas, red bell pepper, cherry tomatoes, red onion, and black olives in a large bowl
2. In a small bowl, whisk together olive oil, red wine vinegar, minced garlic, and oregano
3. Pour dressing over salad and toss to coat evenly
4. Season with salt and pepper

Tips:

- Include crumbled feta cheese for added flavor and protein
- Let the salad marinate for at least 30 minutes before serving to enhance flavors
- Serve over a bed of fresh greens for a more filling meal

Nutritional Values: Calories: 220, Fat: 9g, Carbs: 27g, Protein: 7g, Sugar: 5g, Sodium: 300mg, Potassium: 350mg, Cholesterol: 0mg

TURMERIC TOFU AND KALE STIR-FRY

Preparation Time: 10 min
Cooking Time: 10 min
Servings: 3
Glycemic Index: Low(~48)
Ingredients:

- 1 lb tofu, firm, drained and cubed
- 2 cups kale, chopped
- 1 Tbsp olive oil
- 2 tsp turmeric, ground
- 1 inch ginger, grated
- 2 cloves garlic, minced
- 1 Tbsp soy sauce, low sodium
- 1 Tbsp sesame seeds
- Salt and pepper to taste

Directions:

1. Heat olive oil in a skillet over medium heat
2. Add ginger and garlic, sauté for 2 min
3. Add tofu and turmeric, cook until tofu is golden brown, approximately 5 min
4. Add kale and soy sauce, stir-fry until kale is wilted, about 3 min
5. Garnish with sesame seeds

Tips:

- Serve with cauliflower rice for a complete low-carb meal
- Increase heat for a slightly charred flavor
- Add a splash of lime juice for extra zest

Nutritional Values: Calories: 230, Fat: 14g, Carbs: 12g, Protein: 16g, Sugar: 2g, Sodium: 250mg, Potassium: 350mg, Cholesterol: 0mg

SMOKED SALMON AND CREAM CHEESE CUCUMBER ROLLS

Preparation Time: 15 min
Cooking Time: none
Servings: 4
Glycemic Index: Low(~30)
Ingredients:

- 1 large cucumber, thinly sliced lengthwise
- 4 oz smoked salmon
- 1/4 C. cream cheese, low-fat
- 1 Tbsp chives, chopped
- 1 tsp dill, fresh, chopped
- Pepper to taste

Directions:

1. Lay cucumber slices flat on a clean surface
2. Spread a thin layer of cream cheese on each slice
3. Top with a small piece of smoked salmon
4. Sprinkle with chives and dill
5. Roll each cucumber slice tightly
6. Arrange on a platter and season with pepper

Tips:

- Use a vegetable peeler or mandoline for uniform cucumber slices
- If desired, add a thin strip of avocado inside each roll for extra creaminess
- Chill before serving to firm up the cream cheese slightly

Nutritional Values: Calories: 100, Fat: 6g, Carbs: 4g, Protein: 7g, Sugar: 2g, Sodium: 200mg, Potassium: 180mg, Cholesterol: 15mg

CHILLED ZUCCHINI RIBBON SALAD WITH LEMON AND HERBS

Preparation Time: 15 min
Cooking Time: none
Servings: 2
Glycemic Index: Low(~40)
Ingredients:

- 2 zucchinis, thinly sliced into ribbons
- 1 Tbsp extra virgin olive oil
- Juice of 1 lemon
- 1 tsp lemon zest
- 1/4 C. fresh basil, chopped
- 1/4 C. fresh mint, chopped
- Salt to taste
- Black pepper to taste

Directions:

1. Slice zucchinis into thin ribbons using a vegetable peeler or mandoline
2. In a mixing bowl, combine olive oil, lemon juice, lemon zest, fresh basil, and mint
3. Add zucchini ribbons to the dressing and toss gently to coat
4. Season with salt and black pepper to taste
5. Chill in the refrigerator for 10 min before serving

Tips:

- Opt for young, firm zucchinis for best results
- Lemon zest can be adjusted according to taste preference
- This salad pairs well with grilled chicken or fish for a complete meal

Nutritional Values: Calories: 90, Fat: 7g, Carbs: 7g, Protein: 2g, Sugar: 4g, Sodium: 10mg, Potassium: 512mg, Cholesterol: 0mg

CHILLED CUCUMBER AND DILL SOUP

Preparation Time: 10 min
Cooking Time: none
Servings: 2
Glycemic Index: Low(~45)
Ingredients:

- 2 large cucumbers, peeled and diced
- 1 cup plain Greek yogurt
- 2 cloves garlic, minced
- 2 Tbsp fresh dill, chopped
- 1 Tbsp olive oil
- 1 Tbsp lemon juice
- Salt and pepper to taste
- ½ cup cold water

Directions:

1. Combine diced cucumbers, Greek yogurt, minced garlic, chopped dill, olive oil, lemon juice, salt, pepper, and cold water in a blender
2. Blend until smooth and creamy
3. Chill in the refrigerator for at least 1 hour before serving
4. Garnish with additional dill and cucumber slices just before serving

Tips:

- Chill overnight for enhanced flavors
- For a vegan version, substitute Greek yogurt with coconut yogurt
- Add a small pinch of ground cumin for an extra zing

Nutritional Values: Calories: 135, Fat: 7g, Carbs: 12g, Protein: 6g, Sugar: 6g, Sodium: 50mg, Potassium: 440mg, Cholesterol: 10mg

SPICY LENTIL AND CARROT SOUP

Preparation Time: 15 min
Cooking Time: 15 min
Servings: 4
Glycemic Index: Low(~40)
Ingredients:

- 1 cup red lentils
- 4 cups vegetable broth
- 3 carrots, peeled and diced
- 1 onion, diced
- 2 Tbsp olive oil
- 1 tsp turmeric powder
- 1 tsp cumin powder
- Salt and pepper to taste
- Fresh cilantro for garnish

Directions:

1. Heat olive oil in a large pot over medium heat
2. Add diced onions and cook until translucent
3. Add turmeric and cumin, stir for 1 min
4. Add diced carrots and red lentils, stir to coat
5. Pour in vegetable broth, bring to a boil then simmer for 15 min
6. Season with salt and pepper
7. Blend half the soup for a creamy texture, then recombine
8. Serve garnished with fresh cilantro

Tips:

- Serve with a dollop of Greek yogurt for creaminess
- Adding a squeeze of lemon juice enhances the flavors
- For extra heat, include a diced chili pepper with the onions

Nutritional Values: Calories: 230, Fat: 7g, Carbs: 33g, Protein: 11g, Sugar: 5g, Sodium: 300mg, Potassium: 710mg, Cholesterol: 0mg

APPLE FENNEL WALNUT SALAD

Preparation Time: 10 min
Cooking Time: none
Servings: 4
Glycemic Index: Low(~40)

Ingredients:

- 1 fennel bulb, thinly sliced
- 2 apples, sliced
- ½ cup walnuts, toasted
- 2 Tbsp olive oil
- 1 Tbsp apple cider vinegar
- 1 tsp honey
- Salt and pepper to taste
- Mixed greens for serving

Directions:

1. Combine thinly sliced fennel, sliced apples, and toasted walnuts in a salad bowl
2. In a separate small bowl, whisk together olive oil, apple cider vinegar, honey, salt, and pepper
3. Pour dressing over the salad and toss to coat evenly
4. Serve over a bed of mixed greens

Tips:

- Use a mandoline slicer for evenly thin fennel and apple slices
- Swap walnuts with pecans for a different texture
- Drizzle with a bit more honey if you prefer a sweeter salad

Nutritional Values: Calories: 210, Fat: 15g, Carbs: 18g, Protein: 3g, Sugar: 10g, Sodium: 45mg, Potassium: 410mg, Cholesterol: 0mg

BEETROOT AND GOAT CHEESE ARUGULA SALAD

Preparation Time: 10 min
Cooking Time: none
Servings: 2
Glycemic Index: Medium(~56)
Ingredients:

- 2 medium beetroots, cooked and sliced
- 2 cups arugula
- ¼ cup goat cheese, crumbled
- 2 Tbsp walnuts, chopped
- 1 Tbsp balsamic vinegar
- 1 Tbsp olive oil
- Salt and pepper to taste

Directions:

1. Arrange arugula on plates
2. Top with sliced beetroots, crumbled goat cheese, and chopped walnuts
3. In a small bowl, mix balsamic vinegar, olive oil, salt, and pepper
4. Drizzle the dressing over the salads just before serving

Tips:

- Roast beetroots in advance for a richer flavor
- Add a sprinkle of fresh herbs like parsley or basil for extra freshness
- For a low-fat version, replace goat cheese with feta

Nutritional Values: Calories: 220, Fat: 15g, Carbs: 15g, Protein: 6g, Sugar: 9g, Sodium: 130mg, Potassium: 400mg, Cholesterol: 13mg

CUCUMBER RIBBON SALAD WITH FETA AND MINT

Preparation Time: 10 min
Cooking Time: none
Servings: 2
Glycemic Index: Low(~30)
Ingredients:

- 1 large English cucumber
- 1/2 C. feta cheese, crumbled
- 2 Tbsp fresh mint, finely chopped
- 2 Tbsp extra virgin olive oil
- 1 Tbsp lemon juice
- Salt to taste
- Black pepper, freshly ground

Directions:

1. Using a vegetable peeler, peel long, thin ribbons from the cucumber
2. In a large bowl, combine cucumber ribbons with feta cheese and chopped mint
3. Drizzle with olive oil and lemon juice
4. Season with salt and pepper to taste
5. Toss gently until all components are well-coated

Tips:

- Opt for a light drizzle of oil to keep the salad refreshing
- Add a sprinkle of chili flakes for a spicy kick
- Consider adding thinly sliced red onion for extra zest

Nutritional Values: Calories: 150, Fat: 12g, Carbs: 6g, Protein: 4g, Sugar: 3g, Sodium: 320mg, Potassium: 270mg, Cholesterol: 25mg

HEARTY BEET AND BARLEY SOUP

Preparation Time: 15 min
Cooking Time: 15 min
Servings: 4
Glycemic Index: Low(~40)
Ingredients:

- 1 C. barley, rinsed
- 3 medium beets, peeled and diced
- 1 large carrot, diced
- 1 large onion, chopped
- 2 garlic cloves, minced
- 4 C. vegetable stock
- 1 tsp thyme, dried
- Salt and pepper to taste
- Fresh parsley, chopped for garnish

Directions:

1. In a large pot, sauté onion and garlic until translucent
2. Add beets, carrot, thyme, and barley to the pot and stir for a few minutes
3. Pour in the vegetable stock and bring to a boil
4. Reduce heat and simmer until the barley and beets are tender, about 15 min
5. Season with salt and pepper
6. Garnish with chopped parsley before serving

Tips:

- Consider roasting the beets beforehand for a deeper flavor
- Add a dollop of low-fat sour cream or plain Greek yogurt on top before serving for extra creaminess
- Use fresh thyme if available for a more intense flavor

Nutritional Values: Calories: 180, Fat: 1g, Carbs: 35g, Protein: 6g, Sugar: 9g, Sodium: 300mg, Potassium: 350mg, Cholesterol: 0mg

SPICY LENTIL AND SPINACH SOUP

Preparation Time: 10 min
Cooking Time: 20 min
Servings: 3
Glycemic Index: Low(~35)
Ingredients:

- 1 C. red lentils
- 3 C. water
- 2 C. fresh spinach, chopped
- 1 medium onion, diced
- 1 jalapeno, seeded and finely chopped
- 2 Tbsp olive oil
- 1 tsp cumin seeds
- Salt to taste
- Lemon wedges for serving

Directions:

1. Heat olive oil in a large saucepan over medium heat
2. Add cumin seeds and let them sizzle for a few seconds
3. Add onion and jalapeno, cooking until onion is soft
4. Stir in red lentils and water, bring to a boil, then reduce heat to simmer
5. Cook until lentils are tender, about 20 min
6. Add spinach and cook until wilted
7. Season with salt
8. Serve with a wedge of lemon

Tips:

- Integrate a teaspoon of turmeric for added health benefits and color
- Squeeze lemon just before eating to enhance the flavors
- Serve with a slice of whole-grain bread for a filling meal

Nutritional Values: Calories: 200, Fat: 7g, Carbs: 25g, Protein: 12g, Sugar: 3g, Sodium: 200mg, Potassium: 460mg, Cholesterol: 0mg

AVOCADO CHICKEN SALAD WITH LIME AND CILANTRO

Preparation Time: 10 min
Cooking Time: none
Servings: 2
Glycemic Index: Low(~40)
Ingredients:

- 1 large avocado, ripe and diced
- 1/2 lb cooked chicken breast, shredded
- 1/4 C. cilantro, chopped
- Juice of 1 lime
- Salt and pepper to taste
- 1/4 C. red bell pepper, diced

Directions:

1. In a medium bowl, combine avocado, shredded chicken, red bell pepper, and cilantro
2. Squeeze lime juice over the ingredients
3. Season with salt and pepper to taste
4. Toss gently to mix well

Tips:

- Swap lime juice for lemon if preferred
- Add diced cucumber for extra crunch and freshness
- A sprinkle of chili powder can add a nice heat

Nutritional Values: Calories: 220, Fat: 15g, Carbs: 8g, Protein: 17g, Sugar: 2g, Sodium: 70mg, Potassium: 500mg, Cholesterol: 45mg

THAI CUCUMBER AND PEANUT SALAD

Preparation Time: 15 min
Cooking Time: none
Servings: 4
Glycemic Index: Low(~40)
Ingredients:

- 2 large cucumbers, peeled and thinly sliced
- 1 red bell pepper, thinly sliced
- 1/4 C. fresh cilantro, chopped
- 2 Tbsp green onions, sliced
- 1/4 C. dry-roasted peanuts, chopped
- 1 Tbsp sesame seeds
- Dressing: 2 Tbsp lime juice
- 1 Tbsp fish sauce
- 1 tsp stevia
- 1/2 tsp red pepper flakes

Directions:

1. Combine cucumbers, red bell pepper, cilantro, and green onions in a large bowl
2. In a small bowl, whisk together lime juice, fish sauce, stevia, and red pepper flakes to create the dressing
3. Pour dressing over the salad and toss thoroughly to combine
4. Garnish with chopped peanuts and sesame seeds before serving

Tips:

- For added crunch, refrigerate the salad for about 30 min before serving
- If allergic to peanuts, substitute with crushed roasted almonds or cashews
- To enhance the fusion of flavors, let the salad marinate for an extra 10 min after mixing

Nutritional Values: Calories: 120, Fat: 7g, Carbs: 10g, Protein: 4g, Sugar: 5g, Sodium: 300mg, Potassium: 350mg, Cholesterol: 0mg

TUSCAN BEAN SOUP

Preparation Time: 15 min
Cooking Time: 20 min
Servings: 4
Glycemic Index: Low(~50)
Ingredients:

- 2 Tbsp extra virgin olive oil
- 1 medium yellow onion, diced
- 2 cloves garlic, minced
- 1 large carrot, peeled and diced
- 2 stalks celery, diced
- 4 C. low-sodium vegetable broth
- 1 can (15 oz.) cannellini beans, rinsed and drained
- 1 tsp dried thyme
- 1 tsp dried rosemary
- 2 C. kale, roughly chopped
- Salt and pepper to taste

Directions:

1. Heat olive oil in a large pot over medium heat
2. Add onion and garlic, sauté until onion is translucent, about 5 min
3. Add carrot and celery, cook for 5 min
4. Pour in vegetable broth, bring to a boil
5. Add cannellini beans, thyme, and rosemary, reduce heat to low and simmer for 15 min
6. Stir in kale and cook until wilted, about 5 min
7. Season with salt and pepper, serve hot

Tips:

- Use a mix of kale and spinach for added nutrients
- Add a squeeze of lemon juice before serving to enhance flavors
- Blend half the soup for a creamier texture

Nutritional Values: Calories: 190, Fat: 5g, Carbs: 28g, Protein: 9g, Sugar: 4g, Sodium: 300mg, Potassium: 600mg, Cholesterol: 0mg

MUSHROOM AND BARLEY STEW

Preparation Time: 10 min
Cooking Time: 40 min
Servings: 4
Glycemic Index: Medium(~65)
Ingredients:

- 1 Tbsp olive oil
- 1 lb. cremini mushrooms, sliced
- 1 large onion, chopped
- 2 garlic cloves, minced
- 1 C. pearl barley
- 4 C. low-sodium beef broth
- 1 Tbsp Worcestershire sauce
- 2 Tbsp fresh parsley, chopped
- Salt and black pepper to taste

Directions:

1. Heat olive oil in a large pot over medium-high heat
2. Add mushrooms, onion, and garlic, cook until mushrooms are golden, about 10 min
3. Stir in barley and beef broth, bring to boil
4. Reduce heat and simmer until barley is tender, about 30 min
5. Stir in Worcestershire sauce and parsley, season with salt and pepper, simmer for another 5 min
6. Serve warm

Tips:

- Toast barley before adding to the pot for a nuttier flavor
- Serve with a dollop of Greek yogurt for creaminess
- Add chopped carrots for extra sweetness and texture

Nutritional Values: Calories: 215, Fat: 4g, Carbs: 38g, Protein: 9g, Sugar: 5g, Sodium: 290mg, Potassium: 470mg, Cholesterol: 0mg

SPICED LENTIL AND SWEET POTATO STEW

Preparation Time: 10 min
Cooking Time: 30 min
Servings: 4
Glycemic Index: Low(~52)
Ingredients:

- 1 Tbsp coconut oil
- 1 large onion, diced
- 2 cloves garlic, minced
- 2 tsp ground cumin
- 1 tsp ground coriander
- 1 tsp smoked paprika
- 1 large sweet potato, peeled and cubed
- 1 C. red lentils
- 4 C. low-sodium vegetable broth
- 2 Tbsp tomato paste
- Salt and pepper to taste

Directions:

1. Heat coconut oil in a large pot over medium heat
2. Add onion and garlic, cook until softened, about 5 min
3. Stir in cumin, coriander, and paprika, cook for 1 min
4. Add sweet potato, lentils, vegetable broth, and tomato paste, bring to a simmer
5. Cook until lentils and sweet potatoes are tender, about 20 min
6. Season with salt and pepper, serve warm

Tips:

- Include a handful of chopped kale for extra greens
- Serve with a slice of whole-grain bread for dipping
- Add a splash of lemon juice for a fresh zest

Nutritional Values: Calories: 230, Fat: 3g, Carbs: 42g, Protein: 11g, Sugar: 7g, Sodium: 300mg, Potassium: 710mg, Cholesterol: 0mg

CAULIFLOWER AND CHICKPEA MASALA

Preparation Time: 15 min
Cooking Time: 25 min
Servings: 4
Glycemic Index: Low(~54)

Ingredients:

- 1 Tbsp ghee
- 1 head cauliflower, cut into florets
- 1 can (15 oz.) chickpeas, drained and rinsed
- 1 large onion, finely chopped
- 2 cloves garlic, minced
- 1 Tbsp ginger, grated
- 2 tsp garam masala
- 1 tsp turmeric
- 1 can (14.5 oz.) diced tomatoes
- 1 C. low-sodium vegetable broth
- 2 Tbsp cilantro, chopped

Directions:

1. Heat ghee in a large skillet over medium heat
2. Add onion, garlic, and ginger, cook until onions are soft, about 5 min
3. Stir in garam masala, turmeric, cook for 1 min
4. Add cauliflower, chickpeas, tomatoes, and broth, bring to a boil
5. Reduce heat to low, cover, and simmer until cauliflower is tender, about 20 min
6. Garnish with cilantro, serve warm

Tips:

- Serve over a bed of basmati rice for a hearty meal
- Stir in a spoonful of yogurt to add creaminess
- Sprinkle fresh pomegranate seeds before serving for a burst of sweetness

Nutritional Values: Calories: 210, Fat: 6g, Carbs: 30g, Protein: 9g, Sugar: 9g, Sodium: 280mg, Potassium: 650mg, Cholesterol: 0mg

LENTIL AND SPINACH SOUP

Preparation Time: 10 min
Cooking Time: 25 min
Servings: 6
Glycemic Index: Low(~30)
Ingredients:

- 1 Tbsp olive oil
- 1 onion, chopped
- 2 garlic cloves, minced
- 1 carrot, diced
- 1 stalk celery, diced
- 1 cup dried lentils, rinsed
- 6 cups low-sodium vegetable broth
- 2 cups spinach, chopped
- 1 tsp ground cumin
- Salt and pepper to taste

Directions:

1. Heat olive oil in a large pot over medium heat
2. Add chopped onion, garlic, carrot, and celery, cook until softened, about 5 min.
3. Add rinsed lentils, vegetable broth, and ground cumin
4. Bring to a boil, then reduce heat and simmer for about 20 min., until lentils are tender
5. Stir in chopped spinach and cook until wilted, about 2 min.
6. Season with salt and pepper to taste
7. Serve hot

Tips:

- To enhance the flavor, add a squeeze of fresh lemon juice before serving
- For a creamier texture, blend half the soup before adding the spinach
- Use red lentils for a quicker cooking time

Nutritional Values: Calories: 180, Fat: 4g, Carbs: 24g, Protein: 12g, Sugar: 3g, Sodium: 300mg, Potassium: 470mg, Cholesterol: 0mg

TURKEY AND BARLEY STEW

Preparation Time: 15 min
Cooking Time: 25 min
Servings: 4
Glycemic Index: Low(~48)
Ingredients:

- 1 lb turkey breast, cubed
- 1 C. pearl barley
- 2 carrots, diced
- 2 celery stalks, diced
- 1 onion, chopped
- 4 cups low-sodium chicken broth
- 1 tsp dried thyme
- 2 tsp olive oil
- Salt and pepper to taste

Directions:

1. Heat olive oil in a large pot over medium heat
2. Add cubed turkey and cook until lightly browned
3. Add chopped onion, diced carrots, and celery to the pot and sauté until softened
4. Pour in chicken broth and stir in pearl barley and thyme
5. Bring to a boil, then reduce heat and simmer for 25 min or until barley is tender
6. Season with salt and pepper to taste

Tips:

- Opt for low-sodium chicken broth to manage sodium intake
- Add a splash of lemon juice or a dash of paprika for an extra zing
- Serve with a side of steamed green beans for a complete meal

Nutritional Values: Calories: 330, Fat: 6g, Carbs: 40g, Protein: 28g, Sugar: 3g, Sodium: 120mg, Potassium: 670mg, Cholesterol: 45mg

HEARTY LENTIL SOUP WITH KALE

Preparation Time: 20 min
Cooking Time: 30 min
Servings: 6
Glycemic Index: Low(~42)
Ingredients:

- 1 C. dried lentils, rinsed
- 4 C. vegetable broth
- 2 C. kale, chopped
- 1 large carrot, diced
- 1 onion, diced
- 2 cloves garlic, minced
- 1 tsp cumin
- 2 tsp olive oil
- Salt and pepper to taste

Directions:

1. Heat olive oil in a soup pot over medium heat
2. Sauté onion, garlic, and carrot until the onion is translucent
3. Add lentils and vegetable broth
4. Bring to a boil, then reduce heat to simmer for about 20 min or until lentils are tender
5. Stir in chopped kale and cumin, continue to simmer for 10 more min
6. Season with salt and pepper as per taste

Tips:

- Introduce a sprinkle of chili flakes for a little heat if desired
- Pair with a slice of whole-grain bread for an additional fiber boost
- Use different types of kale like red or dinosaur for visual appeal

Nutritional Values: Calories: 210, Fat: 3g, Carbs: 35g, Protein: 12g, Sugar: 3g, Sodium: 90mg, Potassium: 600mg, Cholesterol: 0mg

DINNER RECIPES: DELIGHTS FOR DIABETICS

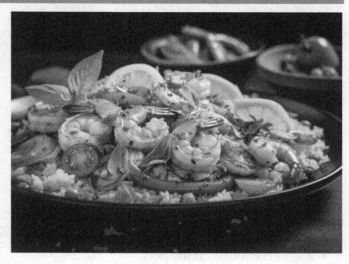

As the sun dips below the horizon and the day's bustle gives way to evening's calm, the dinner table becomes not just a place for eating, but a sanctuary where flavors mingle and memories are made. For those managing diabetes, this meal can seem like a hurdle—another daily challenge in balancing health and satisfaction. Yet, with the right recipes, dinner can transform into a delightful adventure that nurtures both body and spirit.

Imagine a meal that everyone at your table is excited to share; a dish that caters to your dietary needs without feeling restrictive, bringing smiles all around. This isn't just a dream. It's entirely possible and easier than you might think. Here, we explore a range of family-friendly dinners that prove a diabetic diet can be as flavorful and versatile as any other.

The secret lies in understanding the components of your meal. Each recipe in this chapter has been carefully crafted not only to manage blood sugar levels but also to ignite taste buds and offer comfort after a long day. From savory casseroles bursting with color and texture to grilled dishes that bring out hidden aromas and flavors, these meals ensure that every dietary requirement is a pathway to discovery and enjoyment.

Furthermore, each recipe is designed to be straightforward and quick to prepare. Recognizing that evenings are often consumed by work or family activities, these dishes simplify kitchen time without sacrificing quality. You'll find options that can be swiftly assembled with minimal inputs, like a tender, herb-infused chicken that cooks while you unwind, or a robust, veggie-packed stir-fry that comes together in the blink of an eye.

Remember, living with diabetes doesn't mean abandoning the pleasure of meals. On the contrary, it offers an opportunity to reinvent your culinary habits, discovering new favorites while adhering to a health-conscious regimen. Embrace these dinner recipes as your toolkit to not only fuel your body but also to enrich your life, one delicious, wholesome bite at a time. Let's turn dietary management into a celebration of food, health, and togetherness.

CAULIFLOWER RICE STIR-FRY WITH SHRIMP

Preparation Time: 10 min
Cooking Time: 15 min
Servings: 4
Glycemic Index: Low(~50)
Ingredients:

- 1 head cauliflower, grated into 'rice'
- 1 lb shrimp, peeled and deveined
- 2 Tbsp olive oil
- 1 red bell pepper, diced
- 1 cup snap peas, trimmed
- 2 green onions, chopped
- 3 cloves garlic, minced
- 2 Tbsp soy sauce, low sodium
- 1 Tbsp ginger, freshly grated

Directions:

1. Heat olive oil in a large skillet over medium heat
2. Add garlic and ginger, sauté for 1 min until fragrant
3. Increase heat to medium-high, add shrimp and cook until pink, about 3-4 min
4. Remove shrimp and set aside
5. In the same skillet, add grated cauliflower, bell pepper, and snap peas, cook for about 5-6 min until vegetables are tender
6. Return shrimp to the skillet, add soy sauce and green onions, stir well to combine and heat through for about 2 min
7. Serve hot

Tips:

- Consider replacing shrimp with tofu for a vegetarian option
- Add a splash of lime juice for an extra zest
- Include a pinch of chili flakes for a spicy kick

Nutritional Values: Calories: 250, Fat: 10g, Carbs: 18g, Protein: 24g, Sugar: 5g, Sodium: 480mg, Potassium: 700mg, Cholesterol: 180mg

HERBED CHICKEN AND ZUCCHINI SKILLET

Preparation Time: 15 min
Cooking Time: 20 min
Servings: 4
Glycemic Index: Low(~48)
Ingredients:

- 4 skinless boneless chicken breasts
- 2 zucchinis, sliced
- 1 Tbsp olive oil
- 1 tsp rosemary, dried
- 1 tsp thyme, dried
- 2 cloves garlic, minced
- Salt to taste
- Black pepper to taste

Directions:

1. Preheat a skillet over medium heat and add olive oil
2. Season chicken with salt, pepper, rosemary, and thyme
3. Place chicken in the skillet and cook for about 5-6 min on each side until golden and cooked through
4. Remove chicken from skillet and set aside
5. In the same skillet, add minced garlic and zucchini slices, sauté for about 7-8 min until zucchini is tender
6. Return chicken to the skillet, combine with zucchini, and heat through for about 2 min
7. Serve warm

Tips:

- Slice the chicken before serving for easier eating
- Pair this dish with a side of quinoa for additional fiber
- Drizzle with a bit of lemon juice before serving for enhanced flavor

Nutritional Values: Calories: 220, Fat: 6g, Carbs: 8g, Protein: 35g, Sugar: 4g, Sodium: 70mg, Potassium: 800mg, Cholesterol: 80mg

BEEF AND BROCCOLI BOWL WITH CAULIFLOWER MASH

Preparation Time: 20 min
Cooking Time: 25 min
Servings: 4
Glycemic Index: Low(~52)
Ingredients:

- 1 lb lean ground beef
- 2 cups broccoli florets
- 1 head cauliflower, cut into florets
- 1 Tbsp olive oil
- 1 onion, chopped
- 2 cloves garlic, minced
- 2 Tbsp soy sauce, low sodium
- Salt and pepper to taste

Directions:

1. Bring a pot of water to a boil and add cauliflower florets, cook until soft, about 8-10 min
2. Drain and mash cauliflower with a fork or potato masher, set aside
3. Heat olive oil in a skillet over medium-high heat, add garlic and onion, sauté for about 2-3 min until onion is translucent
4. Add ground beef, cook until browned and crumbled, about 7-8 min
5. Add broccoli florets and soy sauce, cover and let steam for about 3-4 min until broccoli is tender but still crisp
6. Serve beef and broccoli over cauliflower mash

Tips:

- Use ground turkey as a leaner alternative to beef
- Add a splash of sesame oil for a nutty flavor
- Garnish with chopped green onions or sesame seeds for an aesthetic touch

Nutritional Values: Calories: 300, Fat: 15g, Carbs: 15g, Protein: 28g, Sugar: 5g, Sodium: 330mg, Potassium: 900mg, Cholesterol: 70mg

SESAME GINGER SALMON WITH SPINACH

Preparation Time: 15 min
Cooking Time: 15 min
Servings: 4
Glycemic Index: Low(~42)
Ingredients:

- 4 salmon fillets, about 6 oz each
- 2 Tbsp sesame oil
- 1 Tbsp ginger, freshly grated
- 3 Tbsp soy sauce, low sodium
- 4 cups spinach, fresh
- 1 Tbsp sesame seeds
- 1 clove garlic, minced

Directions:

1. Preheat oven to 400°F (200°C)
2. In a small bowl, mix sesame oil, soy sauce, grated ginger, and minced garlic
3. Place salmon fillets on a baking sheet lined with parchment paper
4. Pour the sesame-ginger sauce over the salmon fillets and sprinkle with sesame seeds
5. Bake in the oven for about 12-15 min until salmon is cooked through and flakes easily with a fork
6. While salmon is baking, heat a pan over medium-high, add spinach, and sauté until wilted, about 2-3 min
7. Serve the salmon over a bed of sautéed spinach

Tips:

- Add crushed red pepper to the sauce for a spicy contrast
- Combine soy sauce mixture ingredients in advance to save time
- Top with thinly sliced green onions for additional color and flavor

Nutritional Values: Calories: 290, Fat: 15g, Carbs: 8g, Protein: 31g, Sugar: 1g, Sodium: 360mg, Potassium: 850mg, Cholesterol: 60mg

ZUCCHINI AND BELL PEPPER CONFETTI CHICKEN

Preparation Time: 15 min
Cooking Time: 20 min
Servings: 4
Glycemic Index: Low(~40)
Ingredients:

- 1 lb chicken breast, diced
- 1 large zucchini, diced
- 1 red bell pepper, diced
- 1 yellow bell pepper, diced
- 2 cloves garlic, minced
- 1 tsp dried oregano
- 2 Tbsp olive oil
- Salt and pepper to taste

Directions:

1. Preheat oven to 375°F (190°C)
2. In a large skillet, heat olive oil over medium heat
3. Add garlic and sauté until fragrant, about 1 min
4. Add diced chicken breast and cook until golden and nearly cooked through, about 8 min
5. Stir in zucchini, red bell pepper, yellow bell pepper, and oregano
6. Season with salt and pepper
7. Continue to sauté for another 5 min
8. Transfer the skillet contents to a baking dish and bake in the preheated oven for 10 min until vegetables are tender and chicken is fully cooked

Tips:

- For a crispier finish, broil for the last 2 min of baking
- Serve with a side of cauli-rice for an additional low-carb option
- Experiment with varying herbs like basil or thyme for different flavor profiles

Nutritional Values: Calories: 220, Fat: 9g, Carbs: 8g, Protein: 27g, Sugar: 4g, Sodium: 70mg, Potassium: 650mg, Cholesterol: 65mg

CREAMY TURMERIC CAULIFLOWER SOUP

Preparation Time: 10 min
Cooking Time: 20 min
Servings: 4
Glycemic Index: Low(~40)
Ingredients:

- 1 head cauliflower, chopped
- 1 onion, chopped
- 2 cloves garlic, minced
- 3 C. vegetable broth
- 1 tsp turmeric
- 1 tsp ground cumin
- ½ C. coconut milk
- 2 Tbsp olive oil
- Salt and pepper to taste

Directions:

1. In a large pot, heat olive oil over medium heat
2. Add chopped onion and minced garlic, sauté until onion is translucent, about 5 min
3. Stir in turmeric and cumin, cook for 1 min
4. Add chopped cauliflower and vegetable broth, bring to a boil, then reduce heat and simmer until cauliflower is soft, about 15 min
5. Remove from heat, blend the mixture until smooth using an immersion blender
6. Stir in coconut milk and season with salt and pepper
7. Heat through for an additional 2 min, adjusting seasoning if necessary

Tips:

- Serve with a drizzle of olive oil and a sprinkle of fresh parsley for enhanced flavor
- This soup can be stored in the refrigerator for up to 3 days or frozen for a month

Nutritional Values: Calories: 180, Fat: 14g, Carbs: 12g, Protein: 4g, Sugar: 5g, Sodium: 300mg, Potassium: 470mg, Cholesterol: 0mg

LEMON HERB GRILLED SALMON

Preparation Time: 10 min
Cooking Time: 15 min
Servings: 4
Glycemic Index: Low(~35)
Ingredients:

- 4 salmon fillets, about 6 oz each
- 2 lemons, one juiced and one sliced
- 2 Tbsp olive oil
- 1 tsp dried dill
- 1 tsp dried parsley
- Salt and pepper to taste

Directions:

1. Preheat your grill to medium-high heat
2. Mix lemon juice, olive oil, dill, parsley, salt, and pepper in a small bowl to create a marinade
3. Brush both sides of each salmon fillet with the marinade
4. Place lemon slices on the grill and set salmon fillets on top of them
5. Grill the salmon for about 7 min per side or until cooked through and flaky

Tips:

- Pair with a fresh green salad for a full meal
- Keep the skin on the salmon for extra flavor and moisture during grilling
- Avoid flipping the salmon too often to keep it intact

Nutritional Values: Calories: 248, Fat: 14g, Carbs: 3g, Protein: 29g, Sugar: 1g, Sodium: 65mg, Potassium: 830mg, Cholesterol: 75mg

ZUCCHINI AND BASIL PESTO STUFFED CHICKEN

Preparation Time: 15 min
Cooking Time: 20 min
Servings: 4
Glycemic Index: Low(~40)
Ingredients:

- 4 boneless, skinless chicken breasts
- 2 medium zucchinis, grated
- ½ cup basil pesto
- 1 clove garlic, minced
- 2 Tbsp olive oil
- ¼ tsp black pepper
- ¼ cup grated Parmesan cheese
- 1 Tbsp pine nuts

Directions:

1. Preheat oven to 375°F (190°C)
2. Mix zucchini, basil pesto, garlic, Parmesan, and pine nuts in a bowl
3. Cut a pocket in each chicken breast and stuff with zucchini mixture
4. Secure with toothpicks if necessary
5. Brush chicken with olive oil and season with black pepper
6. Bake for 20 min or until chicken is thoroughly cooked

Tips:

- Opt for low-fat pesto to reduce calorie intake
- Keep chicken moist by covering with foil during the first 10 min of baking
- Replace pine nuts with walnuts for a different flavor profile

Nutritional Values: Calories: 290, Fat: 15g, Carbs: 6g, Protein: 28g, Sugar: 2g, Sodium: 320mg, Potassium: 400mg, Cholesterol: 80mg

TURMERIC CAULIFLOWER STEAKS WITH TAHINI DRIZZLE

Preparation Time: 10 min
Cooking Time: 15 min
Servings: 2
Glycemic Index: Low(~35)
Ingredients:

- 1 large head cauliflower, sliced into 1-inch steaks
- 2 Tbsp coconut oil
- 1 tsp turmeric
- ½ tsp cumin
- Salt and black pepper to taste
- 2 Tbsp tahini
- 1 Tbsp lemon juice
- 1 tsp honey
- 1 Tbsp water
- Fresh parsley, chopped

Directions:

1. Preheat oven to 400°F (200°C)
2. Coat cauliflower steaks with coconut oil, turmeric, cumin, salt, and pepper
3. Roast for 15 min, turning once until golden and tender
4. Whisk tahini, lemon juice, honey, and water for the drizzle
5. Serve cauliflower steaks with tahini drizzle and sprinkle with parsley

Tips:

- Substitute honey with a pinch of stevia for a lower sugar option
- Add a sprinkle of chili powder for extra heat
- Ensure cauliflower steaks are cut evenly to cook uniformly

Nutritional Values: Calories: 215, Fat: 15g, Carbs: 18g, Protein: 6g, Sugar: 4g, Sodium: 55mg, Potassium: 470mg, Cholesterol: 0mg

GRILLED SALMON WITH FENNEL AND ORANGE SALAD

Preparation Time: 10 min
Cooking Time: 10 min
Servings: 4
Glycemic Index: Low(~45)
Ingredients:

- 4 salmon fillets, 6 oz each
- 2 fennel bulbs, thinly sliced
- 2 oranges, peeled and segments
- ¼ cup olives, pitted and sliced
- 2 Tbsp olive oil
- Salt and black pepper to taste
- 1 Tbsp dill, fresh and chopped

Directions:

1. Preheat the grill to medium-high
2. Season salmon with salt and black pepper
3. Grill salmon for 5 min on each side or until cooked through
4. Combine fennel, orange segments, olives, and dill in a bowl, drizzle with olive oil, toss gently
5. Serve salmon with fennel and orange salad

Tips:

- Use blood oranges for a vibrant color contrast in the salad
- Brush salmon with a layer of mustard before grilling for additional flavor
- Serve salad chilled for a refreshing taste

Nutritional Values: Calories: 325, Fat: 20g, Carbs: 10g, Protein: 24g, Sugar: 6g, Sodium: 120mg, Potassium: 650mg, Cholesterol: 60mg

SPICY SHRIMP AND BROCCOLI STIR-FRY

Preparation Time: 10 min
Cooking Time: 10 min
Servings: 4
Glycemic Index: Low(~40)
Ingredients:

- 24 large shrimp, peeled and deveined
- 1 head broccoli, cut into florets
- 2 cloves garlic, minced
- 1 inch ginger, grated
- 1 tsp chili flakes
- 2 Tbsp soy sauce, low sodium
- 2 Tbsp sesame oil
- 1 Tbsp lime juice
- Sesame seeds for garnish

Directions:

1. Heat sesame oil in a large pan over medium-high heat
2. Add garlic, ginger, and chili flakes, sauté for 1 min
3. Add broccoli and stir-fry for 5 min
4. Add shrimp, soy sauce, and lime juice, cook until shrimp are pink and cooked through, about 5 min
5. Garnish with sesame seeds

Tips:

- Replace shrimp with tofu for a vegetarian option
- Add a splash of fish sauce for an umami boost
- Incorporate red bell peppers for added color and nutrition

Nutritional Values: Calories: 220, Fat: 10g, Carbs: 8g, Protein: 20g, Sugar: 2g, Sodium: 330mg, Potassium: 300mg, Cholesterol: 115mg

ZESTY LEMON HERB CHICKEN

Preparation Time: 15 min
Cooking Time: 20 min
Servings: 4
Glycemic Index: Low(~40)
Ingredients:

- 4 boneless, skinless chicken breasts
- 2 Tbsp olive oil
- Juice and zest of 1 lemon
- 3 cloves garlic, minced
- 1 tsp dried oregano
- 1 tsp dried thyme
- 1 tsp dried rosemary
- Salt and pepper to taste

Directions:

1. Marinate chicken breasts with olive oil, lemon juice and zest, garlic, oregano, thyme, and rosemary
2. Season with salt and pepper
3. Let marinate for at least 10 min
4. Preheat grill to medium-high (about 375°F/190°C)
5. Grill chicken for about 10 min on each side or until fully cooked and juices run clear

Tips:

- For a charred, smoky flavor, allow chicken to sear for 1-2 min before flipping
- Serve with a side of grilled asparagus or zucchini for a complete meal
- Squeeze extra lemon over cooked chicken for added zest

Nutritional Values: Calories: 210, Fat: 10g, Carbs: 2g, Protein: 29g, Sugar: 1g, Sodium: 65mg, Potassium: 230mg, Cholesterol: 80mg

CAULIFLOWER STEAK WITH WALNUT PESTO

Preparation Time: 10 min
Cooking Time: 15 min
Servings: 2
Glycemic Index: Low(~45)
Ingredients:

- 1 large head cauliflower, sliced into 1-inch steaks
- 2 Tbsp olive oil
- Salt and pepper to taste
- 1/2 cup walnuts
- 1 cup fresh basil leaves
- 2 cloves garlic
- 1/4 cup grated Parmesan cheese
- 1/2 lemon, juiced

Directions:

1. Brush cauliflower steaks with olive oil and season with salt and pepper
2. Roast at 400°F (204°C) for 15 min or until golden and tender
3. Blend walnuts, basil, garlic, Parmesan, and lemon juice to make pesto
4. Serve cauliflower steaks drizzled with walnut pesto

Tips:

- Toast walnuts before blending for deeper flavor
- Replace Parmesan with nutritional yeast for a dairy-free option
- Add chili flakes to pesto for extra spice

Nutritional Values: Calories: 300, Fat: 25g, Carbs: 15g, Protein: 10g, Sugar: 4g, Sodium: 180mg, Potassium: 870mg, Cholesterol: 4mg

SPICED RUBBED SALMON WITH CUCUMBER RELISH

Preparation Time: 10 min
Cooking Time: 15 min
Servings: 4
Glycemic Index: Low(~40)
Ingredients:

- 4 salmon fillets, 6 oz each
- 1 Tbsp chili powder
- 1 tsp cumin
- 1/2 tsp coriander
- 1 cucumber, diced
- 1/4 cup red onion, minced
- 1 jalapeno, minced
- 1/2 cup cilantro, chopped
- Juice of 1 lime
- Salt and pepper to taste

Directions:

1. Mix chili powder, cumin, and coriander and rub onto salmon
2. Preheat oven to 350°F (175°C)
3. Place salmon on a baking sheet and bake for 15 min or until flaky
4. Combine cucumber, red onion, jalapeno, cilantro, lime juice, salt, and pepper to make relish
5. Serve salmon topped with cucumber relish

Tips:

- Avoid overcooking salmon to maintain moisture
- For less heat, remove seeds from jalapeño
- Relish can be made ahead and refrigerated to enhance flavors

Nutritional Values: Calories: 280, Fat: 13g, Carbs: 6g, Protein: 34g, Sugar: 2g, Sodium: 75mg, Potassium: 860mg, Cholesterol: 90mg

HERBED TURKEY AND SPINACH MEATBALLS

Preparation Time: 15 min
Cooking Time: 25 min
Servings: 4
Glycemic Index: Low(~45)
Ingredients:

- 1 lb ground turkey
- 2 cups spinach, finely chopped
- 1/4 cup onion, minced
- 2 cloves garlic, minced
- 1 egg
- 1/4 cup almond flour
- 1 Tbsp Italian herbs
- Salt and pepper to taste

Directions:

1. Combine ground turkey, spinach, onion, garlic, egg, almond flour, and Italian herbs in a bowl
2. Season with salt and pepper
3. Form mixture into golf ball-sized meatballs
4. Place on a baking sheet
5. Preheat oven to 375°F (190°C) and bake for 25 min

Tips:

- Serve with a side of marinara sauce for dipping
- Almond flour can be replaced with crushed flaxseed for an Omega-3 boost
- Add grated zucchini to meatballs for extra moisture

Nutritional Values: Calories: 220, Fat: 12g, Carbs: 4g, Protein: 25g, Sugar: 1g, Sodium: 80mg, Potassium: 320mg, Cholesterol: 100mg

ZUCCHINI NOODLE SHRIMP SCAMPI

Preparation Time: 20 min
Cooking Time: 10 min
Servings: 4
Glycemic Index: Low(~50)
Ingredients:

- 4 zucchinis, spiralized
- 1 lb shrimp, peeled and deveined
- 3 cloves garlic, minced
- 2 Tbsp olive oil
- Juice of 1 lemon
- 1 tsp red pepper flakes
- 1/4 cup parsley, chopped
- Salt to taste

Directions:

1. Heat olive oil in a large skillet over medium heat
2. Add garlic and red pepper flakes, sauté for 1 minute
3. Add shrimp and cook until pink, about 2-3 minutes per side
4. Include spiralized zucchini and lemon juice, cook for an additional 3 minutes
5. Remove from heat, season with salt, and garnish with chopped parsley

Tips:

- Opt for larger shrimp for a quicker cook time and enhanced flavor
- Incorporate a sprinkle of grated Parmesan if not strictly avoiding dairy
- Add cherry tomatoes for a pop of color and a boost of antioxidants

Nutritional Values: Calories: 210, Fat: 8g, Carbs: 10g, Protein: 25g, Sugar: 4g, Sodium: 570mg, Potassium: 510mg, Cholesterol: 180mg

LEMON HERB TILAPIA WITH ZUCCHINI RIBBONS

Preparation Time: 10 min
Cooking Time: 15 min
Servings: 2
Glycemic Index: Low(~40)
Ingredients:

- 2 tilapia fillets
- 2 zucchinis, spiralized into ribbons
- 1 lemon, juiced and zested
- 2 Tbsp olive oil
- 1 tsp dried oregano
- 1 tsp dried basil
- Salt and pepper to taste

Directions:

1. Preheat oven to 375°F (190°C)
2. Lay tilapia fillets and zucchini ribbons on a baking sheet
3. Drizzle with olive oil and lemon juice, then season with lemon zest, oregano, basil, salt, and pepper
4. Bake for 15 min or until fish flakes easily with a fork

Tips:

- For an added flavor boost, top with fresh parsley before serving
- If spiralizing zucchini is not an option, use a vegetable peeler to create thin ribbons
- Squeeze extra lemon over the dish right before eating for a fresher taste

Nutritional Values: Calories: 220, Fat: 10g, Carbs: 6g, Protein: 25g, Sugar: 3g, Sodium: 50mg, Potassium: 400mg, Cholesterol: 60mg

SPICED CHICKEN AND CAULIFLOWER RICE

Preparation Time: 15 min
Cooking Time: 10 min
Servings: 2
Glycemic Index: Low(~50)
Ingredients:

- 2 skinless, boneless chicken breasts, cubed
- 1 cup cauliflower rice
- 1 red bell pepper, diced
- 1 Tbsp coconut oil
- 2 tsp curry powder
- 1 tsp turmeric
- Salt and pepper to taste

Directions:

1. Heat coconut oil in a skillet over medium heat
2. Add chicken cubes and sauté until lightly browned, about 5 min
3. Stir in red bell pepper, curry powder, turmeric, salt, and pepper and continue to sauté for 5 more min
4. Mix in cauliflower rice and cook for another 5 min or until chicken is cooked through and veggies are tender

Tips:

- Experiment with different spice blends like garam masala or cumin for variety
- Serve with a side of lime wedges for a citrusy punch
- Add a splash of coconut milk for a creamier texture

Nutritional Values: Calories: 295, Fat: 12g, Carbs: 8g, Protein: 38g, Sugar: 4g, Sodium: 70mg, Potassium: 500mg, Cholesterol: 95mg

GARLIC SHRIMP WITH ASPARAGUS

Preparation Time: 10 min
Cooking Time: 10 min
Servings: 2
Glycemic Index: Low(~45)
Ingredients:

- 12 large shrimp, peeled and deveined
- 1 bunch of asparagus, trimmed and cut into 1-inch pieces
- 3 cloves garlic, minced
- 1 Tbsp olive oil
- 1 lemon, juiced
- Salt and pepper to taste

Directions:

1. Heat olive oil in a skillet over medium heat
2. Add minced garlic and sauté for 1 min until fragrant
3. Add shrimp and asparagus, season with salt and pepper, and cook for about 7-8 min, or until shrimp are pink and asparagus is tender
4. Drizzle with lemon juice before serving

Tips:

- Serve immediately for best flavor
- For a zestier taste, add a sprinkle of red pepper flakes
- Pair with a small serving of quinoa for those not strictly low-carb

Nutritional Values: Calories: 184, Fat: 8g, Carbs: 5g, Protein: 24g, Sugar: 2g, Sodium: 180mg, Potassium: 300mg, Cholesterol: 180mg

TURMERIC GINGER SALMON

Preparation Time: 15 min
Cooking Time: 15 min
Servings: 2
Glycemic Index: Low(~54)
Ingredients:

- 2 salmon fillets
- 1 Tbsp olive oil
- 1 tsp ground turmeric
- 1 tsp ground ginger
- Salt and pepper to taste
- 1 Tbsp honey (for those who can manage a slight increase in sugars)

Directions:

1. Preheat grill to medium-high heat (375°F or 190°C)
2. Mix olive oil, turmeric, ginger, salt, and pepper, and brush onto salmon fillets
3. Grill salmon for about 6-7 min per side or until cooked through and flaky
4. Drizzle with honey in the last 2 min of cooking for a hint of sweetness

Tips:

- Omit honey if managing very strict sugar intake
- Serve with a side of steamed broccoli or green beans for a complete meal
- Enhance flavor with a squeeze of fresh orange juice over the salmon before serving

Nutritional Values: Calories: 280, Fat: 13g, Carbs: 4g, Protein: 34g, Sugar: 3g (omit if not using honey), Sodium: 75mg, Potassium: 700mg, Cholesterol: 80mg

ZUCCHINI AND BASIL FRITTATA

Preparation Time: 10 min
Cooking Time: 15 min
Servings: 4
Glycemic Index: Low(~40)
Ingredients:

- 6 eggs, whole
- 2 medium zucchini, shredded
- ½ cup fresh basil, chopped
- 1 clove garlic, minced
- ¼ cup Parmesan cheese, grated
- 1 Tbsp olive oil
- Salt to taste
- Pepper to taste

Directions:

1. Preheat oven to 375°F (190°C)
2. Whisk eggs in a large bowl and incorporate shredded zucchini, basil, garlic, and Parmesan cheese
3. Season with salt and pepper
4. Heat olive oil in an oven-safe skillet over medium heat
5. Pour egg mixture into skillet and cook for 3 min without stirring
6. Transfer skillet to oven and bake until eggs are set, about 12 min
7. Slice into wedges and serve hot

Tips:

- Use a well-greased skillet to prevent sticking
- Add a pinch of red pepper flakes for a spicy kick
- Pair with a side salad for a complete meal

Nutritional Values: Calories: 200, Fat: 14g, Carbs: 4g, Protein: 14g, Sugar: 2g, Sodium: 340mg, Potassium: 240mg, Cholesterol: 215mg

LEMON GARLIC SHRIMP WITH ASPARAGUS

Preparation Time: 5 min
Cooking Time: 10 min
Servings: 4
Glycemic Index: Low(~35)
Ingredients:

- 1 lb shrimp, peeled and deveined
- 1 bunch asparagus, trimmed and cut into 1-inch pieces
- 2 Tbsp olive oil
- 3 cloves garlic, minced
- 1 lemon, juiced and zested
- Salt to taste
- Pepper to taste

Directions:

1. Heat olive oil in a large skillet over medium-high heat
2. Add garlic and sauté for 1 min
3. Add asparagus and cook for 4 min
4. Add shrimp and cook until pink and firm, about 3 min
5. Stir in lemon juice and zest
6. Season with salt and pepper
7. Serve immediately

Tips:

- Do not overcook the shrimp to keep them juicy
- Use fresh lemon juice for best flavor
- Garnish with parsley for added freshness

Nutritional Values: Calories: 180, Fat: 8g, Carbs: 5g, Protein: 23g, Sugar: 1g, Sodium: 210mg, Potassium: 300mg, Cholesterol: 180mg

TURMERIC CHICKEN STIR-FRY

Preparation Time: 10 min
Cooking Time: 10 min
Servings: 4
Glycemic Index: Low(~45)
Ingredients:

- 1 lb chicken breast, thinly sliced
- 1 red bell pepper, sliced
- 1 cup broccoli florets
- 1 onion, sliced
- 2 Tbsp coconut oil
- 1 Tbsp turmeric, ground
- 1 tsp ginger, minced
- Salt to taste
- Pepper to taste

Directions:

1. Heat coconut oil in a wok or large skillet over medium-high heat
2. Add onion and sauté for 2 min
3. Add chicken and cook until no longer pink, about 5 min
4. Add bell pepper, broccoli, turmeric, and ginger
5. Stir-fry for another 3 min
6. Season with salt and pepper
7. Serve hot

Tips:

- Cut vegetables in uniform sizes for even cooking
- Sprinkle with sesame seeds for a nutty flavor
- Serve over a bed of cauliflower rice for a complete meal

Nutritional Values: Calories: 220, Fat: 9g, Carbs: 7g, Protein: 29g, Sugar: 3g, Sodium: 200mg, Potassium: 500mg, Cholesterol: 65mg

SPICED PORK TENDERLOIN WITH CAULIFLOWER MASH

Preparation Time: 15 min
Cooking Time: 15 min
Servings: 4
Glycemic Index: Low(~45)
Ingredients:

- 1 pork tenderloin, about 1 lb
- 1 Tbsp paprika
- 1 tsp cumin
- 1 head cauliflower, cut into florets
- 2 Tbsp unsalted butter
- ¼ cup milk, low-fat
- Salt to taste
- Pepper to taste

Directions:

1. Preheat oven to 375°F (190°C)
2. Season pork tenderloin with paprika, cumin, salt, and pepper
3. Roast in the oven until the internal temperature reaches 145°F (63°C), about 15 min
4. Meanwhile, steam cauliflower florets until tender
5. Mash cauliflower with butter and milk until smooth
6. Season with salt and pepper
7. Slice tenderloin and serve with cauliflower mash

Tips:

- Use a meat thermometer to ensure pork is cooked safely
- Add garlic to the cauliflower mash for enhanced flavor
- Let pork rest for 5 min before slicing to retain juices

Nutritional Values: Calories: 240, Fat: 10g, Carbs: 9g, Protein: 30g, Sugar: 4g, Sodium: 220mg, Potassium: 670mg, Cholesterol: 80mg

SHRIMP AND AVOCADO SALAD

Preparation Time: 15 min
Cooking Time: none
Servings: 2
Glycemic Index: Low(~35)
Ingredients:

- 200g shrimps, cooked and peeled
- 1 large avocado, diced
- 1 C. cherry tomatoes, halved
- 1/2 C. cucumber, diced
- 2 Tbsp red onion, finely chopped
- Juice of 1 lime
- 2 Tbsp cilantro, chopped
- Salt and pepper to taste

Directions:

1. Combine all ingredients in a large bowl
2. Toss gently to mix
3. Chill in the refrigerator for 10 min before serving to allow flavors to blend

Tips:

- Use pre-cooked, refrigerated shrimps to save time
- Add a dash of chili flakes for a spicy kick
- Leftovers make a great next-day lunch option

Nutritional Values: Calories: 290, Fat: 15g, Carbs: 12g, Protein: 25g, Sugar: 3g, Sodium: 210mg, Potassium: 450mg, Cholesterol: 180mg

SNACKS AND APPETIZERS: HEALTHY NIBBLES

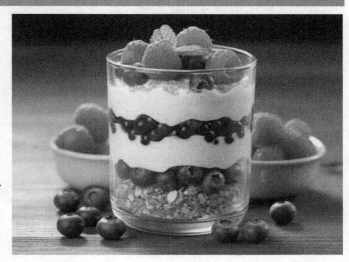

Amidst the bustling rhythm of daily life, we often find ourselves confronted with the sudden pangs of hunger. It's that time, between one significant meal and the next, where a quick, thoughtful nibble can make all the difference in managing both energy and blood sugar levels. Snacks and appetizers, while seemingly modest, play a pivotal role in the daily diet of those managing diabetes or prediabetes, especially over the age of fifty.

Imagine you're in the middle of your day, perhaps returning from a brisk walk or sitting down after sorting the garden, and you feel that familiar stomach rumble. In a world without dietary restrictions, you might reach for anything within arm's length - a sliver of cake, a handful of chips. However, managing diabetes means making smarter, more deliberate choices. This doesn't mean compromising on taste or joy. The trick lies in transforming these quick bites into opportunities for nourishment and delight.

Take for instance a Sunday afternoon: you're hosting friends for a casual get-together, knowing well your need to stick to your diabetic meal plan. Instead of bowls laden with sugary treats or salty, processed snacks, the table is adorned with an array of vibrant, flavorful appetizers. There are stuffed mushrooms, brimming with herbed ricotta, cherry tomatoes broiled with a sprinkle of Parmesan and flakes of sea salt, and mini skewers of olive, feta, and cucumber – each delivering taste without unnecessary sugars or excessive carbs.

In this chapter, we explore how to make such moments of indulgence align perfectly with your health goals. It isn't just about reducing carbs or cutting sugar – it's about reimagining what a snack can be. By incorporating whole, nutrient-rich ingredients, these simple dishes not only satisfy those sudden hunger attacks but also contribute to a balanced diabetic diet.

Re-learning how to snack might seem like a small step, but it's pivotal in transforming your relationship with food. In making every bite count - in both nutrients and pleasure - you set the stage for not just a healthier diet but a joyful, sustainable lifestyle. So as we delve into these recipes, remember, each snack is more than just a quick eat; it's a building block in your life-changing journey towards health and happiness.

CHIA SEED AND COCONUT YOGURT PARFAIT

Preparation Time: 15 min
Cooking Time: none
Servings: 2
Glycemic Index: Low(~35)
Ingredients:
- 1 C. coconut yogurt, unsweetened
- 3 Tbsp chia seeds
- ½ C. mixed berries (blueberries, raspberries)
- 1 Tbsp almond slivers, toasted
- 1 tsp vanilla extract
- 2 tsp coconut flakes, unsweetened

Directions:

1. Mix coconut yogurt with vanilla extract and chia seeds in a bowl and let sit for 10 minutes to allow chia seeds to swell
2. Layer the thickened yogurt mixture with mixed berries in two glasses
3. Top each parfait with toasted almond slivers and coconut flakes
4. Serve chilled

Tips:

- Store in refrigerator overnight for a thicker texture
- Top with a drizzle of almond butter for additional richness
- If berries are not in season, substitute with low-GI fruits like kiwi or peaches

Nutritional Values: Calories: 180, Fat: 9g, Carbs: 18g, Protein: 5g, Sugar: 8g, Sodium: 30mg, Potassium: 150mg, Cholesterol: 0mg

SPICY ROASTED CHICKPEAS

Preparation Time: 10 min
Cooking Time: 20 min
Servings: 4
Glycemic Index: Low(~48)
Ingredients:
- 1 can chickpeas (15 oz.), rinsed and dried
- 1 Tbsp olive oil
- 1 tsp smoked paprika
- ½ tsp cayenne pepper
- ½ tsp garlic powder
- Salt to taste
- ½ tsp black pepper, ground

Directions:

1. Preheat oven to 400°F (200°C)
2. Toss chickpeas with olive oil, smoked paprika, cayenne pepper, garlic powder, salt, and black pepper in a bowl until evenly coated
3. Spread chickpeas on a baking sheet and roast in the oven until crispy, about 20 min
4. Let cool before serving

Tips:

- Omit cayenne pepper for a less spicy version
- Store in an airtight container for up to a week for a crunchy snack on the go
- Experiment with different spices like turmeric or cumin for variety

Nutritional Values: Calories: 134, Fat: 5g, Carbs: 18g, Protein: 6g, Sugar: 0g, Sodium: 200mg, Potassium: 210mg, Cholesterol: 0mg

CUCUMBER ROLL-UPS WITH HUMMUS

Preparation Time: 15 min
Cooking Time: none
Servings: 3
Glycemic Index: Low(~49)
Ingredients:

- 1 large cucumber, thinly sliced lengthwise
- ½ C. hummus
- ¼ C. carrots, grated
- 1 Tbsp parsley, chopped
- 1 tsp lemon zest
- Salt and black pepper to taste

Directions:

1. Lay cucumber slices on a clean surface
2. Spread a thin layer of hummus on each slice
3. Top with grated carrots, chopped parsley, and a sprinkle of lemon zest
4. Carefully roll up the cucumber slices and secure with a toothpick
5. Season with salt and black pepper to taste

Tips:

- Opt for a low-sodium hummus to keep the snack heart-healthy
- Add a small amount of spicy paprika to the hummus for an extra kick
- These roll-ups can be made ahead and stored in the refrigerator for a quick snack

Nutritional Values: Calories: 60, Fat: 2.5g, Carbs: 8g, Protein: 3g, Sugar: 2g, Sodium: 120mg, Potassium: 181mg, Cholesterol: 0mg

ZESTY LIME AND AVOCADO SLICES

Preparation Time: 10 min
Cooking Time: none
Servings: 2
Glycemic Index: Low(~42)
Ingredients:

- 1 avocado, ripe but firm
- 1 lime, juiced
- 1 tsp chili flakes
- 1 Tbsp cilantro, finely chopped
- Salt to taste
- 1 Tbsp onion, finely chopped

Directions:

1. Slice avocado into wedges
2. Squeeze lime juice over avocado slices to prevent browning
3. Season with chili flakes, cilantro, onion, and salt
4. Serve immediately or chill before serving

Tips:

- Use lemon juice if lime is not available
- Sprinkle with toasted sesame seeds for a nutty flavor boost
- Increase or decrease chili flakes according to your preference for spice

Nutritional Values: Calories: 154, Fat: 13g, Carbs: 9g, Protein: 2g, Sugar: 1g, Sodium: 5mg, Potassium: 487mg, Cholesterol: 0mg

CHIA LEMON ZEST BITES

Preparation Time: 15 min
Cooking Time: none
Servings: 6
Glycemic Index: Low(~35)
Ingredients:

- 1 C. chia seeds
- ¼ C. lemon zest
- ½ C. coconut flour
- ¼ C. unsweetened shredded coconut
- 3 Tbsp coconut oil, melted
- 2 Tbsp erythritol
- 1 tsp vanilla extract
- A pinch of salt

Directions:

1. Combine chia seeds, lemon zest, coconut flour, shredded coconut, melted coconut oil, erythritol, vanilla extract, and salt in a mixing bowl
2. Mix thoroughly until the mixture holds together
3. Using a spoon, form the mixture into small balls and place them on a tray
4. Refrigerate for at least 1 hr to set

Tips:

- Add a touch of cinnamon for a warm flavor twist
- Keep bites refrigerated in an airtight container to maintain freshness
- Roll the balls in crushed almonds for extra texture and nutty flavor

Nutritional Values: Calories: 130, Fat: 8g, Carbs: 10g, Protein: 3g, Sugar: 0g, Sodium: 5mg, Potassium: 70mg, Cholesterol: 0mg

SAVORY ALMOND FLAX CRACKERS

Preparation Time: 20 min
Cooking Time: none
Servings: 4
Glycemic Index: Low(~40)
Ingredients:

- ½ C. flaxseed meal
- ½ C. almond flour
- 1 Tbsp dried rosemary
- 1 tsp garlic powder
- ½ tsp sea salt
- ¼ C. water
- 1 Tbsp olive oil

Directions:

1. Mix flaxseed meal, almond flour, dried rosemary, garlic powder, and sea salt in a large bowl
2. Add water and olive oil to the dry ingredients and mix until a dough forms
3. Place the dough between two sheets of parchment paper and roll out to 1/8 inch thick
4. Cut into squares and place on a baking sheet
5. Bake at 350°F (175°C) until crisp, about 15 min

Tips:

- Store in an air-tight container to keep the crackers crisp
- Pair with a low-fat cheese or hummus for extra flavor and protein
- Spice up the recipe by adding chili flakes

Nutritional Values: Calories: 150, Fat: 12g, Carbs: 8g, Protein: 5g, Sugar: 0g, Sodium: 120mg, Potassium: 100mg, Cholesterol: 0mg

CUCUMBER HUMMUS BITES

Preparation Time: 10 min
Cooking Time: none
Servings: 6
Glycemic Index: Low(~35)
Ingredients:

- 1 large cucumber, peeled and thickly sliced
- 1 cup hummus, preferably homemade
- 1 tsp paprika
- 1 Tbsp olive oil
- 1/4 cup red bell pepper, finely diced
- 1 Tbsp fresh parsley, chopped
- 1/3 cup feta cheese, crumbled
- 1 tsp lemon zest

Directions:

1. Slice cucumber into thick rounds, ensuring each is sturdy enough to hold toppings
2. Spread a generous layer of hummus on each cucumber slice
3. Sprinkle paprika evenly over the hummus
4. Top each slice with diced red bell pepper, a sprinkle of feta cheese, and lemon zest
5. Drizzle olive oil over the bites and garnish with fresh parsley
6. Serve immediately or chill until ready to serve

Tips:

- Opt for a lemon-infused olive oil to enhance the freshness
- Parsley can be substituted with dill for a different herby profile
- A sprinkle of black sesame seeds can add a nice texture contrast

Nutritional Values: Calories: 150, Fat: 10g, Carbs: 12g, Protein: 5g, Sugar: 2g, Sodium: 210mg, Potassium: 200mg, Cholesterol: 0mg

CHILI LIME SHRIMP CUPS

Preparation Time: 15 min
Cooking Time: 10 min
Servings: 4
Glycemic Index: Low(~40)
Ingredients:

- 24 large shrimp, peeled and deveined
- 2 Tbsp olive oil
- 1 tsp chili powder
- 1 lime, juiced and zested
- 1 garlic clove, minced
- 12 small Bibb lettuce leaves
- 1 small red bell pepper, finely diced
- 1 small avocado, diced
- 1 Tbsp fresh cilantro, chopped

Directions:

1. Marinate shrimp with olive oil, chili powder, lime juice, lime zest, and minced garlic for 10 min
2. Preheat oven to 375°F (190°C)
3. Arrange shrimp on a baking sheet and bake for 10 min until pink and cooked through
4. Place shrimp in Bibb lettuce, top with red bell pepper, avocado, and cilantro
5. Serve immediately

Tips:

- Opt for wild-caught shrimp for better flavor and sustainability
- Lime zest enhances the freshness, don't skip it!
- For extra heat, add a pinch of cayenne to the marinade

Nutritional Values: Calories: 150, Fat: 8g, Carbs: 5g, Protein: 15g, Sugar: 2g, Sodium: 115mg, Potassium: 300mg, Cholesterol: 110mg

MINI BELL PEPPER NACHOS

Preparation Time: 10 min
Cooking Time: 5 min
Servings: 4
Glycemic Index: Low(~35)
Ingredients:

- 12 mini bell peppers, halved and seeds removed
- 1 cup cooked and shredded chicken breast
- ½ cup cheddar cheese, shredded
- ¼ cup black olives, sliced
- 2 green onions, chopped
- 1 jalapeno, thinly sliced
- 1 Tbsp taco seasoning
- 1 small lime, cut into wedges

Directions:

1. Arrange bell pepper halves on a baking tray
2. Mix shredded chicken with taco seasoning, and distribute evenly on bell pepper halves
3. Sprinkle with cheddar cheese, black olives, and jalapeno slices
4. Broil for 5 min or until cheese is melted and bubbly
5. Garnish with green onions and serve with lime wedges on the side

Tips:

- Substitute chicken with ground turkey for a leaner option
- Adding a dollop of guacamole adds creaminess and healthy fats
- Serve on a platter for an eye-catching presentation

Nutritional Values: Calories: 180, Fat: 12g, Carbs: 5g, Protein: 15g, Sugar: 3g, Sodium: 190mg, Potassium: 230mg, Cholesterol: 45mg

CUCUMBER AVOCADO ROLLS

Preparation Time: 20 min
Cooking Time: none
Servings: 4
Glycemic Index: Low(~30)
Ingredients:

- 1 large cucumber
- 1 ripe avocado, mashed
- 1 Tbsp lemon juice
- 2 Tbsp red onion, finely chopped
- 1 Tbsp dill, fresh and chopped
- Salt and pepper, to taste
- 1 Tbsp capers, for garnish

Directions:

1. Slice cucumber into long, thin strips using a mandoline or vegetable peeler
2. Mix mashed avocado with lemon juice, red onion, dill, salt, and pepper
3. Spread avocado mixture on cucumber strips, roll them up tightly
4. Garnish each roll with capers before serving

Tips:

- Use a seedless cucumber for easier rolling
- If capers are too briny, substitute with diced red bell pepper for a sweet crunch
- Chill rolls before serving for a refreshing appetizer

Nutritional Values: Calories: 80, Fat: 6g, Carbs: 6g, Protein: 2g, Sugar: 1g, Sodium: 75mg, Potassium: 250mg, Cholesterol: 0mg

STUFFED MUSHROOMS WITH HERBED CHEESE

Preparation Time: 15 min
Cooking Time: 15 min
Servings: 4
Glycemic Index: Low(~45)
Ingredients:

- 12 large cremini mushrooms, stems removed
- 1 cup herbed goat cheese
- 2 Tbsp almond meal
- 1 garlic clove, minced
- 2 Tbsp parsley, chopped
- 1 Tbsp olive oil
- Salt and pepper, to taste

Directions:

1. Preheat oven to 375°F (190°C)
2. Mix herbed goat cheese, almond meal, garlic, and parsley with a pinch of salt and pepper
3. Fill mushroom caps with cheese mixture
4. Drizzle with olive oil
5. Bake on a parchment-lined tray for 15 min or until mushrooms are tender and filling is golden

Tips:

- Choose firm mushrooms to avoid them getting too soggy
- Serve immediately, or keep warm until serving for best texture
- Pair with a crisp, dry white wine for an elegant touch

Nutritional Values: Calories: 120, Fat: 9g, Carbs: 4g, Protein: 6g, Sugar: 2g, Sodium: 220mg, Potassium: 300mg, Cholesterol: 15mg

GRILLED ZUCCHINI ROLL-UPS WITH HERBED GOAT CHEESE

Preparation Time: 15 min
Cooking Time: 10 min
Servings: 6
Glycemic Index: Low(~35)
Ingredients:

- 3 zucchini, sliced lengthwise into 1/4 inch thick strips
- 2 Tbsp olive oil
- Salt and pepper to taste
- 6 oz. goat cheese, softened
- 1 Tbsp dill, chopped
- 1 Tbsp basil, chopped
- 1 Tbsp parsley, chopped
- 1 clove garlic, minced

Directions:

1. Brush zucchini strips with olive oil and season with salt and pepper
2. Preheat grill to medium-high and grill zucchini strips until tender and slightly charred, about 3 min per side
3. In a bowl, mix goat cheese with dill, basil, parsley, and garlic
4. Spread herbed goat cheese on each zucchini strip and roll up tightly
5. Serve immediately or chill before serving

Tips:

- Prepare zucchini roll-ups ahead of time and refrigerate for a quick appetizer
- Use flavored goat cheese for an extra twist
- Opt for grilling over direct heat to enhance flavor

Nutritional Values: Calories: 180, Fat: 14g, Carbs: 6g, Protein: 7g, Sugar: 3g, Sodium: 200mg, Potassium: 230mg, Cholesterol: 22mg

CUCUMBER CUPS WITH SMOKED SALMON AND DILL CREAM

Preparation Time: 20 min
Cooking Time: none
Servings: 8
Glycemic Index: Low(~30)
Ingredients:

- 2 large cucumbers
- 8 oz. smoked salmon, finely chopped
- 1/2 C. Greek yogurt
- 1 Tbsp lemon juice
- 2 tsp fresh dill, chopped
- Capers for garnish
- Salt and pepper to taste

Directions:

1. Slice cucumbers into 1 inch thick rounds and hollow out centers using a melon baller
2. In a bowl, combine smoked salmon, Greek yogurt, lemon juice, and dill, season with salt and pepper
3. Spoon salmon mixture into cucumber cups and garnish with capers
4. Serve chilled

Tips:

- Scoop the cucumber cups in advance and fill just before serving to maintain freshness
- Add a drop of hot sauce to the dill cream for a spicy kick
- Garnish with a sprig of dill for a fancy touch

Nutritional Values: Calories: 70, Fat: 2g, Carbs: 3g, Protein: 9g, Sugar: 2g, Sodium: 320mg, Potassium: 138mg, Cholesterol: 8mg

SHRIMP AND AVOCADO COCKTAIL SHOOTERS

Preparation Time: 20 min
Cooking Time: none
Servings: 10
Glycemic Index: Low(~30)
Ingredients:

- 20 medium shrimp, cooked and chilled
- 2 avocados, diced
- 1/2 C. cocktail sauce
- 1 Tbsp lime juice
- 1 tsp horseradish
- 10 small glasses
- Salt and pepper to taste
- Lime wedges for garnish

Directions:

1. Mix diced avocados with lime juice, horseradish, salt, and pepper in a bowl
2. Place a spoonful of avocado mixture at the bottom of each glass
3. Top with cocktail sauce
4. Add two shrimps per glass
5. Garnish with a lime wedge and serve immediately

Tips:

- Prepare in small glasses for elegant presentation
- Swapping horseradish for prepared wasabi can add a fiery twist
- Pre-chill the glasses to keep the cocktail cool longer

Nutritional Values: Calories: 100, Fat: 7g, Carbs: 6g, Protein: 6g, Sugar: 2g, Sodium: 300mg, Potassium: 180mg, Cholesterol: 40mg

CUCUMBER ROLL-UPS WITH HERBED CREAM CHEESE AND SMOKED SALMON

Preparation Time: 15 min
Cooking Time: none
Servings: 6
Glycemic Index: Low(~30)
Ingredients:

- 1 large cucumber, sliced lengthwise into thin strips using a mandoline
- 4 oz cream cheese, softened
- 1 Tbsp dill, freshly chopped
- 1 Tbsp chives, freshly chopped
- 6 oz smoked salmon, thinly sliced
- 1 tsp lemon zest
- 1 Tbsp lemon juice

Directions:

1. Combine cream cheese, dill, chives, lemon zest, and lemon juice in a bowl and mix until smooth
2. Lay cucumber strips flat and spread a thin layer of the herbed cream cheese mixture on each strip
3. Place a small piece of smoked salmon on one end of each cucumber strip
4. Carefully roll up the cucumber strips, starting from the salmon end, forming tight rolls

Tips:

- Ensure cucumber strips are patted dry before applying cream cheese to prevent slipping
- Can substitute smoked salmon with thinly sliced turkey for a different flavor profile
- Prepare a few hours ahead and refrigerate to enhance flavors

Nutritional Values: Calories: 120, Fat: 9g, Carbs: 3g, Protein: 8g, Sugar: 2g, Sodium: 400mg, Potassium: 150mg, Cholesterol: 30mg

CHERRY TOMATOES STUFFED WITH GOAT CHEESE AND HERBS

Preparation Time: 20 min
Cooking Time: none
Servings: 12
Glycemic Index: Low(~35)

Ingredients:

- 24 cherry tomatoes
- 6 oz goat cheese, softened
- 2 Tbsp basil, finely chopped
- 2 Tbsp parsley, finely chopped
- Black pepper, freshly ground
- 1 garlic clove, minced

Directions:

1. Slice the tops off cherry tomatoes and scoop out the insides with a small spoon
2. In a small bowl, mix goat cheese, basil, parsley, minced garlic, and a pinch of black pepper until well combined
3. Carefully stuff the hollowed-out cherry tomatoes with the goat cheese mixture
4. Chill before serving to firm up the cheese stuffing

Tips:

- Use a melon baller to easily scoop out tomato insides without breaking the skin
- For a zesty twist, add a dash of lemon zest to the goat cheese mix
- Cherry tomatoes can be prepped a day in advance and stored in the refrigerator

Nutritional Values: Calories: 50, Fat: 4g, Carbs: 1g, Protein: 3g, Sugar: 1g, Sodium: 65mg, Potassium: 90mg, Cholesterol: 10mg

CHIA AND ALMOND BUTTER ENERGY BALLS

Preparation Time: 15 min
Cooking Time: none
Servings: 8
Glycemic Index: Low(~30)
Ingredients:

- ¼ cup chia seeds
- ½ cup almond butter, unsweetened
- ¼ cup shredded coconut, unsweetened
- 2 Tbsp flaxseeds, ground
- 2 Tbsp cocoa powder, unsweetened
- 1 tsp cinnamon, ground
- ¼ cup erythritol
- 2 tsp vanilla extract

Directions:

1. Combine chia seeds, almond butter, shredded coconut, ground flaxseeds, cocoa powder, cinnamon, erythritol, and vanilla extract in a large bowl
2. Mix thoroughly until all ingredients are well combined and the mixture becomes sticky
3. Using your hands, form the mixture into small balls about the size of a walnut
4. Store in an airtight container in the refrigerator to set for at least 2 hours before serving

Tips:

- For smoother energy balls, blend the mixture in a food processor before forming into balls
- Store these energy balls in the freezer for a chilled treat
- Roll the balls in extra shredded coconut or cocoa powder for an added touch

Nutritional Values: Calories: 150, Fat: 9g, Carbs: 12g, Protein: 4g, Sugar: 1g, Sodium: 20mg, Potassium: 120mg, Cholesterol: 0mg

PEPPERED TURKEY JERKY STRIPS

Preparation Time: 10 min
Cooking Time: 4 hr
Servings: 4
Glycemic Index: Low(~40)
Ingredients:

- 1 lb lean turkey breast, cut into strips
- 2 Tbsp apple cider vinegar
- 1 Tbsp Worcestershire sauce
- 1 tsp black pepper, coarsely ground
- 1 tsp garlic powder
- 1 Tbsp smoked paprika
- 1 Tbsp soy sauce, low sodium
- pinch of stevia

Directions:

1. Mix apple cider vinegar, Worcestershire sauce, black pepper, garlic powder, smoked paprika, soy sauce, and stevia in a bowl to create a marinade
2. Toss turkey strips in the marinade ensuring they are well coated
3. Allow to marinate for 30 min to 2 hr in the refrigerator
4. Preheat oven to 175°F (80°C)
5. Arrange marinated turkey strips on a baking rack over a baking sheet
6. Bake in the oven for about 4 hr or until dried and chewy

Tips:

- Use the lowest temperature setting in your oven to ensure even drying without cooking the turkey strips
- Turn the strips halfway through drying for even dehydration
- Marinate overnight for more pronounced flavors

Nutritional Values: Calories: 110, Fat: 1g, Carbs: 2g, Protein: 20g, Sugar: 0g, Sodium: 75mg, Potassium: 200mg, Cholesterol: 50mg

SAVORY ROASTED CHICKPEAS

Preparation Time: 10 min
Cooking Time: 30 min
Servings: 4
Glycemic Index: Low(~55)
Ingredients:

- 1 can chickpeas, drained and dried
- 1 Tbsp olive oil
- 1 tsp rosemary, dried
- 1 tsp thyme, dried
- ½ tsp salt, optional
- ¼ tsp black pepper, ground
- 1 tsp onion powder
- 1 tsp garlic powder

Directions:

1. Preheat oven to 400°F (200°C)
2. In a bowl, toss drained chickpeas with olive oil, rosemary, thyme, optional salt, black pepper, onion powder, and garlic powder until evenly coated
3. Spread chickpeas on a baking sheet in a single layer
4. Roast in the oven for 30 min, stirring occasionally, until crisp and golden

Tips:

- For extra crispiness, leave the chickpeas in the oven after turning it off for an additional 10 min to cool slowly
- Experiment with different spices like smoked paprika or cumin for variety
- Ensure chickpeas are thoroughly dried before roasting for the best texture

Nutritional Values: Calories: 120, Fat: 5g, Carbs: 15g, Protein: 5g, Sugar: 3g, Sodium: 300mg if salt used, Potassium: 170mg, Cholesterol: 0mg

SPICED PEAR CHIPS

Preparation Time: 10 min
Cooking Time: 2 hr
Servings: 2
Glycemic Index: Low(~35)
Ingredients:

- 2 large pears, thinly sliced
- 1 tsp ground cinnamon
- ¼ tsp ground nutmeg
- 1 Tbsp lemon juice
- ¼ tsp stevia

Directions:

1. In a bowl, toss thinly sliced pears with lemon juice, cinnamon, nutmeg, and stevia until evenly coated
2. Arrange slices in a single layer on a baking sheet lined with parchment paper
3. Preheat oven to 225°F (105°C)
4. Bake for 2 hr, flipping halfway through, until the pear chips are crisp and dry

Tips:

- Slice pears as thinly and uniformly as possible for even baking
- After baking, let the pear chips cool in the oven to enhance their crispiness
- Store in an airtight container to maintain freshness

Nutritional Values: Calories: 80, Fat: 0g, Carbs: 20g, Protein: 0g, Sugar: 12g, Sodium: 0mg, Potassium: 100mg, Cholesterol: 0mg

ZESTY LEMON RICOTTA BITES

Preparation Time: 10 min
Cooking Time: none
Servings: 4
Glycemic Index: Low(~35)
Ingredients:

- 1 cup ricotta cheese, part-skim
- 1 lemon, zest and juice
- 2 Tbsp chives, finely chopped
- ¼ tsp black pepper, freshly ground
- Pinch of salt
- 8 slices cucumber, thick-cut
- 4 tsp almond slivers, toasted

Directions:

1. Combine ricotta cheese, lemon zest, lemon juice, chives, black pepper, and a pinch of salt in a bowl
2. Mix thoroughly to blend all ingredients
3. Spoon the ricotta mixture onto cucumber slices and garnish with toasted almond slivers
4. Serve chilled

Tips:

- Incorporate herbs like dill or mint for a fresh flavor twist
- For a crunchier base, use sliced bell peppers instead of cucumber
- The mixture can be made in advance and refrigerated overnight for enhanced flavors

Nutritional Values: Calories: 100, Fat: 7g, Carbs: 4g, Protein: 5g, Sugar: 2g, Sodium: 60mg, Potassium: 100mg, Cholesterol: 15mg

SMOKY PAPRIKA CHICKPEA POPCORN

Preparation Time: 15 min
Cooking Time: none
Servings: 2
Glycemic Index: Low(~48)
Ingredients:

- 1 can chickpeas, drained and patted dry
- 1 Tbsp olive oil
- 1 tsp smoked paprika
- ¼ tsp garlic powder
- Pinch of cayenne pepper
- Salt to taste
- 1 tsp parsley, dried

Directions:

1. Toss chickpeas with olive oil, smoked paprika, garlic powder, cayenne pepper, and salt until evenly coated
2. Spread chickpeas on a baking sheet and toast under the broiler for 10-12 min, shaking the pan occasionally until crispy
3. Sprinkle with dried parsley before serving

Tips:

- Offer a vegan option by substituting with avocado oil
- Can be stored in an airtight container for up to a week for a quick snack
- Adjust the amount of cayenne for desired spiciness

Nutritional Values: Calories: 190, Fat: 6g, Carbs: 28g, Protein: 8g, Sugar: 5g, Sodium: 300mg, Potassium: 350mg, Cholesterol: 0mg

ROSEMARY BEEF CROSTINIS

Preparation Time: 20 min
Cooking Time: 10 min
Servings: 6
Glycemic Index: Low(~45)
Ingredients:

- 12 thin slices whole-grain baguette
- 2 Tbsp olive oil
- 6 oz roast beef, thinly sliced
- 1 Tbsp rosemary, fresh, chopped
- ¼ cup red onion, thinly sliced
- 1 Tbsp balsamic glaze
- Black pepper to taste

Directions:

1. Preheat oven to 350°F (175°C)
2. Brush baguette slices with olive oil and toast in the oven until crisp, about 10 min
3. Top each slice with roast beef, a sprinkle of chopped rosemary, and a few slices of red onion
4. Drizzle with balsamic glaze and season with black pepper
5. Serve immediately

Tips:

- Experiment with different herbs like thyme or basil for variety
- Use a low sodium roast beef to keep salt intake in check
- Balsamic reduction can be used instead of glaze for a more profound flavor

Nutritional Values: Calories: 120, Fat: 5g, Carbs: 10g, Protein: 10g, Sugar: 1g, Sodium: 180mg, Potassium: 200mg, Cholesterol: 25mg

SPICY EDAMAME DIP

Preparation Time: 10 min
Cooking Time: none
Servings: 3
Glycemic Index: Low(~32)
Ingredients:

- 1 cup edamame, cooked and shelled
- 1 garlic clove, minced
- 2 Tbsp tahini
- 1 Tbsp lemon juice
- ¼ tsp chili flakes
- Salt to taste
- 1 Tbsp olive oil

Directions:

1. Combine edamame, garlic, tahini, lemon juice, chili flakes, and salt in a food processor
2. Process until smooth, gradually adding olive oil until the desired consistency is achieved
3. Serve chilled with vegetable sticks or whole-grain crackers

Tips:

- Adjust the amount of chili flakes based on spice preference
- Try adding a small piece of avocado for creaminess and a dose of healthy fats
- Leftover dip can be spread on sandwiches or wraps for an extra protein boost

Nutritional Values: Calories: 150, Fat: 10g, Carbs: 9g, Protein: 8g, Sugar: 1g, Sodium: 100mg, Potassium: 300mg, Cholesterol: 0mg

SATISFYING THE SWEET TOOTH: DESSERT RECIPES

Imagine a world where indulging your sweet tooth doesn't have to mean veering off your nutritional path. For many managing diabetes or prediabetes, the thought of dessert invokes a wave of guilt—almost a forbidden fruit in the realm of dietary restrictions. But what if I told you that savoring a rich, sweet dessert could still be part of your health journey? It's not only possible; it's a delightful reality we're going to explore in this chapter.

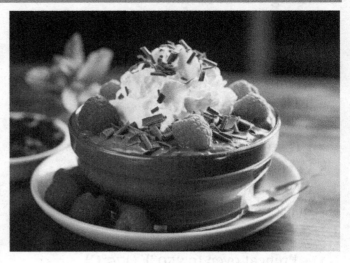

Through the pages to follow, we'll delve into the art of creating decadent desserts that align beautifully with your dietary needs. You won't find any sugar-laden, carb-heavy recipes here. Instead, I'll introduce you to a variety of treats crafted with low-glycemic sweeteners, nutrient-dense flours, and healthy fats that won't spike your blood sugar levels. Each recipe is designed to bring joy and indulgence back to your dessert plate without compromising your health.

Let's challenge the typical narrative that dessert is a dieter's downfall. With the right ingredients and techniques, your post-meal treats can transform into health-enhancing delicacies. Imagine biting into a silky chocolate mousse, its richness derived from dark cocoa and avocados, sweetened just right with a touch of natural sweetener. Or picture enjoying a slice of fresh berry tart, where the crisp, nutty crust perfectly complements the tart sweetness of ripe, antioxidant-rich berries.

Each dessert you'll discover here is so much more than a mere end to a meal—it's a celebration of flavor and a testament to how our dietary choices can actually enhance our wellbeing. Whether it's a no-bake treat you need in a pinch or a special concoction for a festive occasion, these dessert recipes provide the perfect finale to any meal.

As you embark on this sweet culinary journey, remember that managing diabetes or prediabetes doesn't mean denying yourself the joys of eating. It means adapting, experimenting, and ultimately finding delight in the flavors that also nourish your body.

CHIA CHOCOLATE PUDDING

Preparation Time: 15 min
Cooking Time: none
Servings: 4
Glycemic Index: Low(~30)
Ingredients:

- 1 cup unsweetened almond milk
- 1/3 cup chia seeds
- 1/4 cup unsweetened cocoa powder
- 2 Tbsp erythritol
- 1/2 tsp vanilla extract
- 1/4 tsp cinnamon, ground
- Pinch of sea salt

Directions:

1. Combine almond milk, chia seeds, cocoa powder, erythritol, vanilla extract, cinnamon, and sea salt in a mixing bowl
2. Whisk thoroughly until well blended
3. Let the mixture sit for 10 min to allow chia seeds to swell
4. Give it another stir and refrigerate for at least 4 hours or overnight until it achieves a pudding-like consistency
5. Stir well before serving

Tips:

- Serve with a dollop of whipped coconut cream for added luxury
- Sprinkle with a touch of flaky sea salt to enhance the chocolate flavor
- Add a few raspberries for a fresh, tart contrast

Nutritional Values: Calories: 135, Fat: 8g, Carbs: 15g, Protein: 4g, Sugar: 1g, Sodium: 60mg, Potassium: 200mg, Cholesterol: 0mg

ALMOND BUTTER FUDGE SQUARES

Preparation Time: 20 min
Cooking Time: 1 hr chilling
Servings: 12
Glycemic Index: Low(~35)
Ingredients:

- 1 cup almond butter, smooth
- 1/4 cup coconut oil, melted
- 2 Tbsp coconut flour
- 1 Tbsp erythritol
- 1 tsp vanilla extract
- 1/4 tsp sea salt

Directions:

1. Mix almond butter, melted coconut oil, coconut flour, erythritol, vanilla extract, and sea salt in a bowl until combined
2. Pour the mixture into a parchment-lined square baking dish
3. Spread evenly using a spatula
4. Refrigerate for at least 1 hr or until set
5. Cut into squares

Tips:

- Store in the refrigerator in an airtight container to maintain freshness
- For a nuttier flavor, roast the almond butter slightly before use
- Try adding chopped nuts or seeds for added texture and nutrients

Nutritional Values: Calories: 180, Fat: 16g, Carbs: 6g, Protein: 4g, Sugar: 1g, Sodium: 75mg, Potassium: 210mg, Cholesterol: 0mg

COCONUT LEMON BARS

Preparation Time: 10 min
Cooking Time: 25 min
Servings: 8
Glycemic Index: Low(~40)
Ingredients:

- 1/2 cup coconut flour
- 1/4 cup erythritol
- 1/4 cup unsweetened shredded coconut
- 1/4 cup coconut oil, melted
- 3 large eggs
- 1/4 cup lemon juice, fresh
- 1 Tbsp lemon zest
- 1/2 tsp vanilla extract

Directions:

1. Preheat oven to 350°F (175°C)
2. Combine coconut flour, erythritol, and shredded coconut in a mixing bowl
3. Stir in melted coconut oil until a crumbly dough forms
4. Press this dough evenly into a greased 8x8 inch baking dish
5. Bake for 10 min
6. Whisk eggs, lemon juice, lemon zest, and vanilla together
7. Pour over the baked crust
8. Return to oven and bake for an additional 15 min or until set
9. Cool before cutting into bars

Tips:

- Add a sprinkle of powdered erythritol on top for a sweet finish
- Pair with a scoop of sugar-free vanilla ice cream for a decadent dessert experience
- Increase lemon zest for a more intense lemon flavor

Nutritional Values: Calories: 160, Fat: 12g, Carbs: 8g, Protein: 4g, Sugar: 1g, Sodium: 100mg, Potassium: 75mg, Cholesterol: 70mg

AVOCADO COCOA MOUSSE

Preparation Time: 10 min
Cooking Time: none
Servings: 2
Glycemic Index: Low(~35)
Ingredients:

- 1 ripe avocado
- 1/4 cup unsweetened cocoa powder
- 1/4 cup almond milk
- 2 Tbsp erythritol
- 1 tsp vanilla extract
- Pinch of sea salt

Directions:

1. Peel and pit the avocado
2. Place avocado, cocoa powder, almond milk, erythritol, vanilla extract, and a pinch of sea salt in a blender
3. Blend on high until smooth and creamy
4. Transfer to serving dishes and chill in the fridge until ready to serve

Tips:

- Garnish with a few mint leaves for a refreshing touch
- Mix in a spoonful of peanut butter for a richer flavor
- Serve chilled for the best texture and taste experience

Nutritional Values: Calories: 200, Fat: 15g, Carbs: 17g, Protein: 3g, Sugar: 1g, Sodium: 75mg, Potassium: 487mg, Cholesterol: 0mg

ZESTY LEMON RICOTTA CHEESECAKE

Preparation Time: 10 min
Cooking Time: 40 min
Servings: 8
Glycemic Index: Low(~45)
Ingredients:

- 15 oz. ricotta cheese, part-skim
- 2 large eggs
- ¾ cup almond flour
- ¼ cup erythritol
- Zest of 1 lemon
- 1 tsp vanilla extract
- 2 Tbsp slivered almonds
- Pinch of salt

Directions:

1. Preheat oven to 325°F (163°C)
2. In a mixing bowl, combine ricotta cheese, eggs, almond flour, erythritol, lemon zest, and vanilla extract
3. Beat until smooth
4. Pour into a greased 9-inch pie pan
5. Sprinkle slivered almonds on top and a pinch of salt
6. Bake for 40 min or until center is set
7. Let cool before serving

Tips:

- Opt for fresh lemon zest to enhance the tangy flavor
- Store in the refrigerator to maintain freshness
- Serve chilled for best taste

Nutritional Values: Calories: 190, Fat: 15g, Carbs: 8g, Protein: 8g, Sugar: 2g, Sodium: 120mg, Potassium: 90mg, Cholesterol: 55mg

SPICED AVOCADO CHOCOLATE MOUSSE

Preparation Time: 15 min
Cooking Time: none
Servings: 4
Glycemic Index: Low(~40)
Ingredients:

- 1 ripe avocado
- 1/4 cup unsweetened cocoa powder
- 1/4 cup almond milk
- 2 Tbsp monk fruit sweetener
- 1/2 tsp ground cinnamon
- 1/4 tsp chili powder
- 1 tsp vanilla extract

Directions:

1. Combine avocado, cocoa powder, almond milk, monk fruit sweetener, cinnamon, chili powder, and vanilla extract in a blender
2. Blend until smooth and creamy
3. Divide into serving dishes
4. Refrigerate for at least 1 hr before serving

Tips:

- Add a dollop of coconut cream for extra richness
- Sprinkle a pinch of sea salt before serving to enhance flavors
- For a milder taste, adjust chili powder according to preference

Nutritional Values: Calories: 140, Fat: 10g, Carbs: 12g, Protein: 2g, Sugar: 1g, Sodium: 20mg, Potassium: 370mg, Cholesterol: 0mg

ALMOND COCONUT TRUFFLES

Preparation Time: 20 min
Cooking Time: none
Servings: 12
Glycemic Index: Low(~45)
Ingredients:

- 1 cup shredded coconut, unsweetened
- ½ cup almond meal
- ¼ cup coconut oil, melted
- 3 Tbsp erythritol
- 1 tsp vanilla extract
- ⅛ tsp sea salt
- Extra shredded coconut for rolling

Directions:

1. Mix shredded coconut, almond meal, melted coconut oil, erythritol, vanilla extract, and sea salt in a bowl until well combined
2. Shape the mixture into small balls
3. Roll each ball in extra shredded coconut to coat
4. Chill in the refrigerator for 20 min before serving

Tips:

- Store in an airtight container in the fridge to keep fresh for up to a week
- Roll in cocoa powder instead of coconut for a chocolate version
- Use a cookie scoop for uniform truffles

Nutritional Values: Calories: 130, Fat: 12g, Carbs: 4g, Protein: 2g, Sugar: 1g, Sodium: 30mg, Potassium: 50mg, Cholesterol: 0mg

BERRY CHIA PUDDING PARFAIT

Preparation Time: 15 min
Cooking Time: none
Servings: 4
Glycemic Index: Low(~47)
Ingredients:

- 2 cups unsweetened almond milk
- ½ cup chia seeds
- 1 Tbsp monk fruit sweetener
- 1 tsp vanilla extract
- 1 cup mixed berries (raspberries, blueberries, strawberries), fresh
- Mint leaves for garnish

Directions:

1. Mix almond milk, chia seeds, monk fruit sweetener, and vanilla extract in a bowl
2. Stir thoroughly to combine
3. Let sit for 5 min, then stir again to prevent clumping
4. Refrigerate for at least 2 hrs
5. Layer chilled chia pudding with fresh mixed berries in serving glasses
6. Garnish with mint leaves

Tips:

- Stir the chia mixture every few minutes within the first 20 min to ensure even gelling
- Top with toasted coconut flakes for added texture
- Use a blend of seasonal berries for variation

Nutritional Values: Calories: 150, Fat: 9g, Carbs: 15g, Protein: 4g, Sugar: 5g, Sodium: 30mg, Potassium: 200mg, Cholesterol: 0mg

CHIA AND COCONUT RICE PUDDING

Preparation Time: 15 min
Cooking Time: 20 min
Servings: 4
Glycemic Index: Low(~52)
Ingredients:

- 1 C. brown rice, cooked
- 2 C. unsweetened almond milk
- ¼ C. chia seeds
- ¼ C. shredded coconut, unsweetened
- 1 tsp vanilla extract
- 2 Tbsp erythritol
- ½ tsp cinnamon, ground

Directions:

1. Combine almond milk, cooked brown rice, chia seeds, shredded coconut, and erythritol in a large saucepan over medium heat
2. Stir continuously until the mixture begins to simmer
3. Reduce heat to low, add vanilla extract and cinnamon, and simmer for 20 min., stirring occasionally until thickened
4. Remove from heat and cool slightly before serving

Tips:

- Serve warm or chilled
- Top with a sprinkle of cinnamon or nutmeg for extra flavor
- For a creamier texture, blend half of the pudding before adding chia seeds

Nutritional Values: Calories: 215, Fat: 9g, Carbs: 30g, Protein: 5g, Sugar: 1g, Sodium: 50mg, Potassium: 150mg, Cholesterol: 0mg

COCONUT AND ALMOND NO-BAKE COOKIES

Preparation Time: 10 min
Cooking Time: none
Servings: 12
Glycemic Index: Low(~35)
Ingredients:

- 1 cup unsweetened shredded coconut
- 1 cup almond flour
- ½ cup coconut oil, melted
- ⅓ cup erythritol
- 1 tsp vanilla extract
- Pinch of salt

Directions:

1. Combine unsweetened shredded coconut, almond flour, melted coconut oil, erythritol, vanilla extract, and a pinch of salt in a mixing bowl
2. Stir the ingredients vigorously until the mixture is well combined and holds together when squeezed
3. Spoon out the mixture and press firmly to form cookies placed on a parchment-lined tray
4. Chill in the refrigerator to set for about 20 minutes before serving

Tips:

- Use a cookie scoop for even size and presentation
- Store in the refrigerator in an airtight container for up to a week
- Press a whole almond on top of each cookie before chilling for added texture and flavor

Nutritional Values: Calories: 150, Fat: 14g, Carbs: 4g, Protein: 2g, Sugar: 1g, Sodium: 10mg, Potassium: 0mg, Cholesterol: 0mg

RASPBERRY CHIA SEED PUDDING

Preparation Time: 15 min
Cooking Time: none
Servings: 4
Glycemic Index: Low(~30)
Ingredients:

- 1 cup unsweetened almond milk
- ½ cup chia seeds
- 1 cup raspberries, fresh
- 2 Tbsp erythritol
- 1 tsp vanilla extract

Directions:

1. Combine unsweetened almond milk, chia seeds, erythritol, and vanilla extract in a bowl
2. Mix thoroughly until the chia seeds start to swell and the mixture becomes gelatinous
3. Gently fold in fresh raspberries
4. Divide the mixture into serving dishes and refrigerate for at least 3 hours to allow the pudding to set

Tips:

- Serve with a sprinkle of crushed almonds for added crunch
- If fresh raspberries are unavailable, thawed frozen raspberries can substitute well
- Adjust sweetness by altering the amount of erythritol according to taste

Nutritional Values: Calories: 130, Fat: 8g, Carbs: 12g, Protein: 4g, Sugar: 2g, Sodium: 30mg, Potassium: 150mg, Cholesterol: 0mg

PEANUT BUTTER AND CHOCOLATE HEMP SQUARES

Preparation Time: 20 min
Cooking Time: none
Servings: 8
Glycemic Index: Low(~40)
Ingredients:

- ¾ cup natural peanut butter
- ¼ cup hemp seeds
- ¼ cup cocoa powder, unsweetened
- ½ cup coconut oil, melted
- 1 Tbsp erythritol
- ¼ tsp salt

Directions:

1. Mix natural peanut butter, unsweetened cocoa powder, melted coconut oil, erythritol, and salt in a bowl until smooth
2. Stir in hemp seeds for texture
3. Pour the mixture into a lined square dish and smooth with a spatula
4. Refrigerate until firm, about 1 hr, then cut into squares

Tips:

- Store squares in the fridge to maintain texture
- Swap hemp seeds for chia seeds if preferred for a variation in texture
- Drizzle melted dark chocolate over the top for added indulgence before chilling

Nutritional Values: Calories: 200, Fat: 18g, Carbs: 8g, Protein: 6g, Sugar: 1g, Sodium: 100mg, Potassium: 200mg, Cholesterol: 0mg

LEMON CASHEW DATE BARS

Preparation Time: 15 min
Cooking Time: none
Servings: 10
Glycemic Index: Low(~40)
Ingredients:

- 1 cup dates, pitted
- 1 cup cashews, raw
- ½ cup unsweetened shredded coconut
- 2 Tbsp coconut oil
- 1 lemon, zest and juice
- ¼ tsp vanilla extract

Directions:

1. Place pitted dates, raw cashews, unsweetened shredded coconut, coconut oil, zest and juice of one lemon, and vanilla extract in a food processor
2. Process until the mixture is sticky and holds together
3. Press the mixture into a lined pan and chill in the refrigerator to harden
4. Slice into bars

Tips:

- Roll individual bars in extra shredded coconut for a decorative finish
- Keep bars chilled until serving to maintain their shape
- Add a pinch of sea salt to enhance the sweet and tart flavors from the dates and lemon

Nutritional Values: Calories: 180, Fat: 12g, Carbs: 18g, Protein: 3g, Sugar: 14g, Sodium: 5mg, Potassium: 250mg, Cholesterol: 0mg

ALMOND COCONUT ENERGY BALLS

Preparation Time: 15 min
Cooking Time: none
Servings: 10
Glycemic Index: Low(~35)
Ingredients:

- 1 cup almonds, finely ground
- ½ cup unsweetened shredded coconut
- ¼ cup coconut oil, melted
- 1 tsp vanilla extract
- 3 Tbsp monk fruit sweetener
- 2 Tbsp chia seeds
- 1 pinch sea salt

Directions:

1. Combine ground almonds, shredded coconut, melted coconut oil, vanilla extract, monk fruit sweetener, chia seeds, and sea salt in a large bowl
2. Mix thoroughly until the mixture is well combined and sticky
3. Scoop out the mixture and roll into small balls, about 1 inch in diameter
4. Refrigerate for 10 min to set the energy balls

Tips:

- Store in an airtight container in the fridge for up to a week for best freshness
- Roll balls in additional shredded coconut before setting for extra texture and flavor
- If mixture is too dry, add a bit more melted coconut oil to help binding

Nutritional Values: Calories: 130, Fat: 11g, Carbs: 4g, Protein: 3g, Sugar: 1g, Sodium: 5mg, Potassium: 75mg, Cholesterol: 0mg

NO-BAKE PEANUT BUTTER OAT BARS

Preparation Time: 20 min
Cooking Time: none
Servings: 12
Glycemic Index: Low(~40)
Ingredients:

- 1 cup natural peanut butter, smooth
- 2 cups rolled oats
- ¼ cup flaxseed, ground
- 6 Tbsp erythritol
- ½ cup dark chocolate chips, sugar-free
- 1 tsp cinnamon, ground
- ¼ cup almond milk, unsweetened

Directions:

1. Mix peanut butter, rolled oats, ground flaxseed, erythritol, dark chocolate chips, and ground cinnamon in a large mixing bowl
2. Add almond milk gradually and stir until the mixture becomes consistent and holds together
3. Press the mixture into a lined 8x8 inch pan and chill in the refrigerator for 15 min to firm up

Tips:

- Cut into bars before fully set to make slicing easier
- Can be stored in the refrigerator for up to two weeks, or frozen for longer shelf life
- Substitute almond butter for peanut butter for a different flavor profile

Nutritional Values: Calories: 200, Fat: 14g, Carbs: 15g, Protein: 6g, Sugar: 1g, Sodium: 10mg, Potassium: 180mg, Cholesterol: 0mg

AVOCADO LIME CHEESECAKE CUPS

Preparation Time: 30 min
Cooking Time: none
Servings: 8
Glycemic Index: Low(~30)
Ingredients:

- 2 medium avocados, ripe and peeled
- 1 cup cream cheese, light
- ¼ cup lime juice, fresh
- 1 Tbsp lime zest
- 3 Tbsp monk fruit sweetener
- 1 vanilla bean, seeds scraped
- ½ cup almond flour for crust
- 3 Tbsp coconut oil, melted

Directions:

1. Prepare crust by mixing almond flour with melted coconut oil in a bowl until crumbly
2. Press the crust mixture into the bottoms of small cupcake liners or molds
3. Blend avocados, light cream cheese, lime juice, lime zest, monk fruit sweetener, and vanilla bean seeds until smooth
4. Spoon the avocado mixture over the crust in each mold
5. Chill in the fridge for at least 20 min to set the cheesecake cups

Tips:

- Garnish with additional lime zest or thin lime slices for a refreshing twist
- Use a food processor or blender to ensure the filling is creamy and smooth
- If desired, swap lime juice and zest for lemon for a different citrus flavor

Nutritional Values: Calories: 180, Fat: 15g, Carbs: 8g, Protein: 4g, Sugar: 1g, Sodium: 60mg, Potassium: 250mg, Cholesterol: 15mg

CINNAMON WALNUT FIG BITES

Preparation Time: 20 min
Cooking Time: none
Servings: 15
Glycemic Index: Low(~38)
Ingredients:

- 1 cup walnuts, finely chopped
- 1 cup dried figs, stems removed and finely chopped
- 2 Tbsp coconut flour
- 1 tsp cinnamon, ground
- 2 Tbsp almond butter
- 1 Tbsp chia seeds
- 2 Tbsp water, as needed

Directions:

1. Combine finely chopped walnuts, dried figs, coconut flour, ground cinnamon, almond butter, and chia seeds in a large mixing bowl
2. Add water slowly and mix until the ingredients stick together and can be formed easily
3. Shape the mixture into small balls, roughly 1 inch in diameter
4. Chill in the refrigerator for about 10 min to firm up the bites

Tips:

- These bites can be customized with different nuts or seeds for varied flavors
- Excellent as a grab-and-go snack or an after-meal treat
- If figs are too dry, soak them in warm water for 10 min before chopping

Nutritional Values: Calories: 100, Fat: 7g, Carbs: 9g, Protein: 2g, Sugar: 6g, Sodium: 2mg, Potassium: 108mg, Cholesterol: 0mg

COCONUT & ALMOND ENERGY BALLS

Preparation Time: 15 min
Cooking Time: none
Servings: 10
Glycemic Index: Low(~35)
Ingredients:

- 1 cup unsweetened shredded coconut
- ½ cup almond flour
- ¼ cup coconut oil, melted
- 3 Tbsp monk fruit sweetener
- 1 tsp vanilla extract
- pinch of salt

Directions:

1. Combine unsweetened shredded coconut, almond flour, melted coconut oil, monk fruit sweetener, vanilla extract, and a pinch of salt in a mixing bowl
2. Mix thoroughly until the mixture is well combined and sticks together
3. Shape the mixture into 1-inch balls and place on a parchment paper-lined tray
4. Chill in the refrigerator until firm, about 10-15 minutes

Tips:

- Store in a cool, dry place for up to a week for best freshness
- Roll in cocoa powder or crushed nuts for extra flavor and texture
- Press the center of each ball and add a dollop of almond butter for a creamy surprise

Nutritional Values: Calories: 130, Fat: 11g, Carbs: 5g, Protein: 2g, Sugar: 1g, Sodium: 10mg, Potassium: 85mg, Cholesterol: 0mg

KIWI LIME SORBET

Preparation Time: 10 min
Cooking Time: none
Servings: 4
Glycemic Index: Low(~50)
Ingredients:

- 3 kiwis, peeled and pureed
- Juice of 2 limes
- 2 cups water
- 1 Tbsp erythritol
- 1 tsp fresh mint, finely chopped

Directions:

1. Combine kiwi puree, lime juice, water, and erythritol in a large bowl and mix thoroughly
2. Pour the mixture into an ice cream maker and churn according to the manufacturer's instructions until it reaches a sorbet consistency
3. Fold in the chopped mint and freeze until set
4. Serve chilled

Tips:

- Opt for organic kiwis to enhance the flavor and nutritional benefits
- Mint can be substituted with basil for a different herbal note
- To intensify sweetness without extra erythritol, concentrate the lime juice by simmering it briefly before cooling and adding to the mix

Nutritional Values: Calories: 90, Fat: 0.3g, Carbs: 22g, Protein: 1g, Sugar: 12g, Sodium: 5mg, Potassium: 210mg, Cholesterol: 0mg

BAKED CINNAMON APPLE CHIPS

Preparation Time: 5 min
Cooking Time: 2 hr 30 min
Servings: 4
Glycemic Index: Low(~34)
Ingredients:

- 2 large apples, thinly sliced
- 1 tsp cinnamon
- 1 Tbsp stevia

Directions:

1. Preheat oven to 200°F (93°C)
2. Arrange apple slices in a single layer on a baking sheet lined with parchment paper
3. Sprinkle cinnamon and stevia evenly over the apple slices
4. Bake for 2 hours, turning halfway through, until the apple slices are crisp
5. Allow to cool completely before serving

Tips:

- Use a mandolin slicer for uniformly thin apple slices, which ensures even baking
- Experiment with different apple varieties for varied sweetness levels and textures
- Store in an airtight container to maintain crispness

Nutritional Values: Calories: 50, Fat: 0g, Carbs: 13g, Protein: 0g, Sugar: 10g, Sodium: 2mg, Potassium: 100mg, Cholesterol: 0mg

RASPBERRY PEACH GELATIN CUPS

Preparation Time: 15 min
Cooking Time: 4 hr (chilling time)
Servings: 6
Glycemic Index: Low(~30)
Ingredients:

- 2 cups raspberries, fresh
- 2 peaches, diced
- 2 cups water
- 1 Tbsp agar-agar powder
- 1 tsp lemon juice
- 1 Tbsp monk fruit sweetener

Directions:

1. Combine water, agar-agar, and monk fruit sweetener in a saucepan and bring to a simmer, stirring until the agar-agar is completely dissolved
2. Remove from heat and stir in lemon juice
3. Fold in fresh raspberries and diced peaches
4. Pour mixture into individual serving cups and refrigerate until set, about 4 hours
5. Serve chilled

Tips:

• Opt for ripe but firm peaches for the best texture in the gelatin

• Agar-agar can be found in most health food stores and provides a plant-based alternative to traditional gelatin

• Garnish with a sprig of mint for added freshness and a pop of color

Nutritional Values: Calories: 35, Fat: 0.2g, Carbs: 8g, Protein: 0.5g, Sugar: 4g, Sodium: 12mg, Potassium: 90mg, Cholesterol: 0mg

MANGO COCONUT FROZEN YOGURT

Preparation Time: 15 min
Cooking Time: 6 hr (freezing time)
Servings: 4
Glycemic Index: Low(~35)
Ingredients:

- 1 large mango, peeled and diced
- 2 cups Greek yogurt, unsweetened
- 1 Tbsp coconut flakes, unsweetened
- 1 Tbsp erythritol
- Juice of 1 lime

Directions:

1. Blend mango, Greek yogurt, erythritol, and lime juice in a food processor until smooth
2. Stir in coconut flakes
3. Pour the mixture into a freezer-safe container and freeze, stirring every hour to incorporate air and prevent ice crystals, for about 6 hours until firm
4. Serve with additional coconut flakes sprinkled on top

Tips:

• Greek yogurt can be substituted with coconut yogurt for a dairy-free version

• To enhance the tropical flavor, mix in a small amount of pineapple puree

• Ensure to stir frequently during the freezing process to achieve a creamy texture

Nutritional Values: Calories: 120, Fat: 2g, Carbs: 18g, Protein: 8g, Sugar: 16g, Sodium: 30mg, Potassium: 200mg, Cholesterol: 10mg

CHIA AND RASPBERRY PUDDING

Preparation Time: 10 min
Cooking Time: none
Servings: 2
Glycemic Index: Low(~35)
Ingredients:

- 1 C. unsweetened almond milk
- ¼ C. chia seeds
- 1 tsp vanilla extract
- 1 Tbsp erythritol
- ½ C. raspberries, fresh
- Mint leaves for garnish

Directions:

1. Combine unsweetened almond milk, chia seeds, vanilla extract, and erythritol in a bowl
2. Stir thoroughly to mix all ingredients, ensuring there are no clumps
3. Gently fold in fresh raspberries
4. Refrigerate for at least 4 hrs or overnight to let the pudding thicken
5. Garnish with mint leaves before serving

Tips:

- To enhance flavor, add a pinch of ground cinnamon
- For a crunchier texture, top with slivered almonds before serving
- Increase sweetness naturally with a few drops of stevia if desired

Nutritional Values: Calories: 150, Fat: 9g, Carbs: 15g, Protein: 4g, Sugar: 1g, Sodium: 50mg, Potassium: 150mg, Cholesterol: 0mg

PEACH BASIL SORBET

Preparation Time: 15 min
Cooking Time: 2 hrs freezing time
Servings: 4
Glycemic Index: Low(~40)
Ingredients:

- 2 C. peaches, peeled and diced
- 1 Tbsp fresh basil, chopped
- 1 Tbsp lemon juice
- ½ C. water
- 2 Tbsp monk fruit sweetener

Directions:

1. Blend peaches, fresh basil, lemon juice, water, and monk fruit sweetener in a blender until smooth
2. Pour mixture into a shallow dish and freeze for 1 hr
3. Stir the mixture and return to freezer
4. Freeze until solid, approximately 1 additional hr
5. Serve immediately or store in an airtight container in the freezer

Tips:

- For a smoother texture, blend the mixture again before the final freezing
- Add a splash of sparkling water before serving for a fizzy twist
- Garnish with extra basil leaves for added aroma

Nutritional Values: Calories: 70, Fat: 0.5g, Carbs: 17g, Protein: 1g, Sugar: 15g, Sodium: 1mg, Potassium: 190mg, Cholesterol: 0mg

BLUEBERRY LIME DRIZZLE

Preparation Time: 8 min
Cooking Time: none
Servings: 2
Glycemic Index: Low(~40)
Ingredients:

- 1 C. blueberries, fresh
- Juice of 2 limes
- 1 tsp lime zest
- 1 Tbsp erythritol
- Mint leaves for garnish
- Crushed ice

Directions:

1. Mash fresh blueberries and mix with lime juice, lime zest, and erythritol in a bowl until well combined
2. Serve over crushed ice in glasses
3. Garnish with mint leaves

Tips:

- Experiment with different berries like strawberries for variety
- For extra sweetness, add a little more erythritol to taste
- Serve immediately for freshest flavor

Nutritional Values: Calories: 50, Fat: 0.3g, Carbs: 12g, Protein: 0.7g, Sugar: 7g, Sodium: 2mg, Potassium: 85mg, Cholesterol: 0mg

KIWI COCONUT TARTLETS

Preparation Time: 15 min
Cooking Time: none
Servings: 6
Glycemic Index: Low(~40)
Ingredients:

- 6 kiwis, peeled and sliced
- 1 C. shredded coconut, unsweetened
- ½ C. almond flour
- ¼ C. coconut oil, melted
- 1 tsp vanilla extract
- 2 Tbsp erythritol

Directions:

1. Combine shredded coconut, almond flour, melted coconut oil, vanilla extract, and erythritol in a bowl and mix until a dough forms
2. Press the mixture into small tart molds
3. Arrange kiwi slices on top of each tart base
4. Chill in the refrigerator for at least 2 hrs before serving

Tips:

- Try topping with a dollop of Greek yogurt for extra creaminess
- To add crunch, sprinkle chopped nuts over the kiwi before refrigerating
- Store in an airtight container in the fridge for up to 3 days

Nutritional Values: Calories: 180, Fat: 15g, Carbs: 13g, Protein: 2g, Sugar: 6g, Sodium: 5mg, Potassium: 230mg, Cholesterol: 0mg

A 49-DAY MEAL PLAN

Embarking on a journey to manage diabetes or prediabetes is akin to plotting a course through unknown terrain. It requires a map, a well-stocked supply of necessities, and a steadfast determination. This is where the 49-Day Meal Plan comes into play—an essential part of your navigation toolkit, designed meticulously to guide you step-by-step, meal-by-meal, towards a healthier lifestyle without sacrificing the joys of eating well.

Imagine easing into your mornings with a warm bowl of cinnamon-spiced oatmeal, sweetened naturally and paired with a creamy dollop of Greek yogurt—each component selected not just for its tantalizing flavors but for its ability to regulate your blood sugar. Or visualize a lunch that transports you to a Mediterranean seaside café, despite the simplicity of its preparation. These aren't just meals; they are your allies in your quest for health.

This meal plan is your companion, designed thoughtfully to consider your busy schedule and varying energy levels throughout the day. It appreciates that some evenings are rushed, and offers solutions like quick stir-fries that dance with flavors using fresh herbs and spices instead of relying on processed ingredients. It understands that weekends might allow for more time in the kitchen, suggesting more elaborate dinners that can double as enjoyable family cooking activities.

As we advance through these seven weeks, each recipe and meal combination has been chosen not only for its nutritional value but for its practicality and ease of preparation. From hearty soups that can be batch-cooked and frozen for convenience to vibrant salads that ensure freshness and zest in every bite, this meal plan doesn't just instruct; it inspires.

Step into this journey with confidence, knowing that each meal is a building block towards a healthier you. You'll discover that managing diabetes or prediabetes doesn't require sacrificing flavor or enjoyment—it's about making informed, tasteful choices that delight both the palate and the body. This 49-day guide isn't just about counting carbs or avoiding sugar—it's about rediscovering the pleasure of eating well, with health as a joyful companion on your culinary adventures.

WEEK 1	breakfast	snack	lunch	snack	dinner
Monday	Smoked Salmon and Avocado Wrap	Chili Lime Shrimp Cups	Spicy Lentil and Spinach Soup	Peppered Turkey Jerky Strips	Cauliflower Steak with Walnut Pesto
Tuesday	Spinach and Feta Breakfast Wraps	Cucumber Avocado Rolls	Avocado Chicken Salad with Lime and Cilantro	Shrimp and Avocado Cocktail Shooters	Spiced Rubbed Salmon with Cucumber Relish
Wednesday	Almond Butter and Banana Toast	Savory Almond Flax Crackers	Thai Cucumber and Peanut Salad	Chili Lime Shrimp Cups	Herbed Turkey and Spinach Meatballs
Thursday	Zucchini and Goat Cheese Frittata	Cucumber Hummus Bites	Tuscan Bean Soup	Almond Butter and Banana Open Sandwich	Zucchini Noodle Shrimp Scampi
Friday	Almond Flour Blueberry Pancakes	Savory Roasted Chickpeas	Mushroom and Barley Stew	Grilled Zucchini Roll-Ups with Herbed Goat Cheese	Lemon Herb Tilapia with Zucchini Ribbons
Saturday	Shakshuka with Spinach and Feta	Spinach and Feta Breakfast Wrap	Spiced Lentil and Sweet Potato Stew	Savory Almond Flax Crackers	Spiced Chicken and Cauliflower Rice
Sunday	Coconut Yogurt Parfait with Kiwi and Walnuts	Zucchini Ricotta Pancakes	Cauliflower and Chickpea Masala	Spicy Roasted Chickpeas	Garlic Shrimp with Asparagus

WEEK 2	breakfast	snack	lunch	snack	dinner
Monday	Ricotta and Chive Cloud Pancakes	Zesty Lemon Ricotta Bites	Hearty Turkey and White Bean Chili	Almond Butter and Banana Open Sandwich	Turmeric Ginger Salmon
Tuesday	Mushroom and Spinach Frittata	Savory Roasted Chickpeas	Lentil and Spinach Soup	Stuffed Mushrooms with Herbed Cheese	Zucchini and Basil Frittata
Wednesday	Almond and Coconut Flour Waffles	Peppered Turkey Jerky Strips	Asian Shrimp and Snow Pea Stir-Fry	Spiced Pear Chips	Lemon Garlic Shrimp with Asparagus
Thursday	Savory Yogurt Bowl with Roasted Veggies	Spicy Roasted Chickpeas	Turkey and Barley Stew	Shrimp and Avocado Cocktail Shooters	Turmeric Chicken Stir-Fry
Friday	Savory Spinach and Feta Muffins	Cinnamon Almond Flax Pancakes	Hearty Lentil Soup with Kale	Cucumber Roll-Ups with Hummus	Spiced Pork Tenderloin with Cauliflower Mash
Saturday	Smoked Salmon and Avocado Wrap	Almond Butter and Banana Open Sandwich	Hearty Beet and Barley Soup	Cucumber Avocado Rolls	Shrimp and Avocado Salad
Sunday	Spinach and Feta Breakfast Wraps	Smoky Paprika Chickpea Popcorn	Spicy Lentil and Spinach Soup	Cucumber Roll-Ups with Herbed Cream Cheese and Smoked Salmon	Zesty Lemon Herb Chicken

WEEK 3	breakfast	snack	lunch	snack	dinner
Monday	Almond Butter and Banana Toast	Chia and Almond Butter Energy Balls	Avocado Chicken Salad with Lime and Cilantro	Cucumber Hummus Bites	Cauliflower Steak with Walnut Pesto
Tuesday	Zucchini and Goat Cheese Frittata	Turmeric Pepita Trail Mix	Thai Cucumber and Peanut Salad	Savory Almond Flax Crackers	Spiced Rubbed Salmon with Cucumber Relish
Wednesday	Almond Flour Blueberry Pancakes	Stuffed Mushrooms with Herbed Cheese	Tuscan Bean Soup	Stuffed Mushrooms with Herbed Cheese	Herbed Turkey and Spinach Meatballs
Thursday	Shakshuka with Spinach and Feta	Smoky Paprika Chickpea Popcorn	Mushroom and Barley Stew	Chili Lime Shrimp Cups	Zucchini Noodle Shrimp Scampi
Friday	Coconut Yogurt Parfait with Kiwi and Walnuts	Zesty Lime and Avocado Slices	Spiced Lentil and Sweet Potato Stew	Cucumber Roll-Ups with Hummus	Lemon Herb Tilapia with Zucchini Ribbons
Saturday	Ricotta and Chive Cloud Pancakes	Mini Bell Pepper Nachos	Cauliflower and Chickpea Masala	Chia Seed and Coconut Yogurt Parfait	Spiced Chicken and Cauliflower Rice
Sunday	Mushroom and Spinach Frittata	Cucumber Roll-Ups with Hummus	Spiced Lentil Soup with Spinach	Cucumber Cups with Smoked Salmon and Dill Cream	Garlic Shrimp with Asparagus

WEEK 4	breakfast	snack	lunch	snack	dinner
Monday	Almond and Coconut Flour Waffles	Grilled Zucchini Roll-Ups with Herbed Goat Cheese	Lentil and Spinach Soup	Cucumber Roll-Ups with Herbed Cream Cheese and Smoked Salmon	Turmeric Ginger Salmon
Tuesday	Savory Yogurt Bowl with Roasted Veggies	Peppered Turkey Jerky Strips	Chilled Avocado Soup with Lime and Cilantro	Cucumber Hummus Bites	Zucchini and Basil Frittata
Wednesday	Savory Spinach and Feta Muffins	Spicy Edamame Dip	Turkey and Barley Stew	Zesty Lime and Avocado Slices	Lemon Garlic Shrimp with Asparagus
Thursday	Smoked Salmon and Avocado Wrap	Mini Bell Pepper Nachos	Hearty Lentil Soup with Kale	Spicy Roasted Chickpeas	Turmeric Chicken Stir-Fry
Friday	Spinach and Feta Breakfast Wraps	Cherry Tomatoes Stuffed with Goat Cheese and Herbs	Hearty Beet and Barley Soup	Zesty Lemon Ricotta Bites	Spiced Pork Tenderloin with Cauliflower Mash
Saturday	Almond Butter and Banana Toast	Savory Roasted Chickpeas	Spicy Lentil and Spinach Soup	Shrimp and Avocado Cocktail Shooters	Shrimp and Avocado Salad
Sunday	Zucchini and Goat Cheese Frittata	Chia Lemon Zest Bites	Avocado Chicken Salad with Lime and Cilantro	Turmeric Pepita Trail Mix	Zesty Lemon Herb Chicken

WEEK 5	breakfast	snack	lunch	snack	dinner
Monday	Almond Flour Blueberry Pancakes	Stuffed Mushrooms with Herbed Cheese	Thai Cucumber and Peanut Salad	Rosemary Beef Crostinis	Cauliflower Steak with Walnut Pesto
Tuesday	Shakshuka with Spinach and Feta	Smoky Paprika Chickpea Popcorn	Tuscan Bean Soup	Turmeric Pepita Trail Mix	Spiced Rubbed Salmon with Cucumber Relish
Wednesday	Coconut Yogurt Parfait with Kiwi and Walnuts	Zesty Lime and Avocado Slices	Mushroom and Barley Stew	Savory Almond Flax Crackers	Herbed Turkey and Spinach Meatballs
Thursday	Ricotta and Chive Cloud Pancakes	Cucumber Roll-Ups with Herbed Cream Cheese and Smoked Salmon	Spiced Lentil and Sweet Potato Stew	Spinach and Feta Breakfast Wrap	Zucchini Noodle Shrimp Scampi
Friday	Mushroom and Spinach Frittata	Mini Bell Pepper Nachos	Cauliflower and Chickpea Masala	Zesty Lime and Avocado Slices	Lemon Herb Tilapia with Zucchini Ribbons
Saturday	Almond and Coconut Flour Waffles	Turmeric Pepita Trail Mix	Mediterranean Chickpea Salad	Cucumber Hummus Bites	Spiced Chicken and Cauliflower Rice
Sunday	Savory Yogurt Bowl with Roasted Veggies	Zesty Lemon Ricotta Bites	Lentil and Spinach Soup	Spiced Pear Chips	Garlic Shrimp with Asparagus

WEEK 6	breakfast	snack	lunch	snack	dinner
Monday	Savory Spinach and Feta Muffins	Chia Seed and Coconut Yogurt Parfait	Turmeric Tofu and Kale Stir-Fry	Chia Lemon Zest Bites	Turmeric Ginger Salmon
Tuesday	Smoked Salmon and Avocado Wrap	Rosemary Beef Crostinis	Turkey and Barley Stew	Cherry Tomatoes Stuffed with Goat Cheese and Herbs	Zucchini and Basil Frittata
Wednesday	Spinach and Feta Breakfast Wraps	Spicy Roasted Chickpeas	Hearty Lentil Soup with Kale	Cucumber Avocado Rolls	Lemon Garlic Shrimp with Asparagus
Thursday	Almond Butter and Banana Toast	Chili Lime Shrimp Cups	Hearty Beet and Barley Soup	Spicy Edamame Dip	Turmeric Chicken Stir-Fry
Friday	Zucchini and Goat Cheese Frittata	Spicy Edamame Dip	Spicy Lentil and Spinach Soup	Cherry Tomatoes Stuffed with Goat Cheese and Herbs	Spiced Pork Tenderloin with Cauliflower Mash
Saturday	Almond Flour Blueberry Pancakes	Cucumber Cups with Smoked Salmon and Dill Cream	Avocado Chicken Salad with Lime and Cilantro	Chia Seed and Coconut Yogurt Parfait	Shrimp and Avocado Salad
Sunday	Shakshuka with Spinach and Feta	Cucumber Roll-Ups with Hummus	Thai Cucumber and Peanut Salad	Spiced Pear Chips	Zesty Lemon Herb Chicken

WEEK 7	breakfast	snack	lunch	snack	dinner
Monday	Coconut Yogurt Parfait with Kiwi and Walnuts	Chia Seed and Coconut Yogurt Parfait	Tuscan Bean Soup	Chia and Almond Butter Energy Balls	Cauliflower Steak with Walnut Pesto
Tuesday	Ricotta and Chive Cloud Pancakes	Mini Bell Pepper Nachos	Mushroom and Barley Stew	Cucumber Cups with Smoked Salmon and Dill Cream	Spiced Rubbed Salmon with Cucumber Relish
Wednesday	Mushroom and Spinach Frittata	Grilled Zucchini Roll-Ups with Herbed Goat Cheese	Spiced Lentil and Sweet Potato Stew	Cucumber Cups with Smoked Salmon and Dill Cream	Herbed Turkey and Spinach Meatballs
Thursday	Almond and Coconut Flour Waffles	Rosemary Beef Crostinis	Cauliflower and Chickpea Masala	Chia and Almond Butter Energy Balls	Zucchini Noodle Shrimp Scampi
Friday	Savory Yogurt Bowl with Roasted Veggies	Cucumber Roll-Ups with Herbed Cream Cheese and Smoked Salmon	Smoked Salmon and Cream Cheese Cucumber Rolls	Shrimp and Avocado Cocktail Shooters	Lemon Herb Tilapia with Zucchini Ribbons
Saturday	Savory Spinach and Feta Muffins	Chia Lemon Zest Bites	Lentil and Spinach Soup	Chia Lemon Zest Bites	Spiced Chicken and Cauliflower Rice
Sunday	Smoked Salmon and Avocado Wrap	Grilled Zucchini Roll-Ups with Herbed Goat Cheese	Chilled Zucchini Ribbon Salad with Lemon and Herbs	Cucumber Avocado Rolls	Garlic Shrimp with Asparagus

BEYOND THE DIET: LIFESTYLE AND MINDSET

When we embark on a journey to manage diabetes through diet, it's like setting the stage for a play where nutrition is the star. But the supporting roles—our daily habits, emotional well-being, and the environment we create around us—are equally pivotal in ensuring the performance is a resounding success.

Embarking on this path means more than just choosing the right foods; it's about shaping a lifestyle that supports those choices day after day. Many of us find this idea daunting, especially after a lifetime of different habits. However, embracing healthy changes as a holistic way of living rather than a series of restrictions can transform our approach.

Let's consider the scenario of Sandra, a vibrant 62-year-old recently diagnosed with prediabetes. Like many, the news initially felt like a sentence to a life of bland food and rigorous limitations. But soon, Sandra realized it was a beacon guiding her towards a healthier, more fulfilling way of living. By integrating gentle exercise routines, like morning walks and yoga, into her diet regimen, she didn't just address her blood sugar levels; she also discovered newfound energy and a more positive outlook on life.

Furthermore, cultivating a mindfulness practice helped Sandra remain present during meals, savoring each bite, and recognizing the signals of fullness her body communicated, thus avoiding overeating—a common challenge many face. These small shifts in mindset and lifestyle were not just about managing her prediabetes; they became acts of self-care that nourished her body and soul.

By viewing diet as one key ingredient in a larger recipe for wellness, you, like Sandra, can find greater success and satisfaction. Managing diabetes or prediabetes doesn't end with what's on your plate. It's equally about what you do between meals and how you think and feel about your body and health.

This fuller, richer approach to health can turn the daily management of diabetes into a more enjoyable and sustainable practice. After all, a life well-lived is a tapestry woven from threads of multiple hues and textures, all of which need to harmonize for the most vivid picture.

MANAGING STRESS AND EMOTIONAL EATING

For many managing diabetes or prediabetes, the challenge isn't just tracking carbs or reading food labels—the emotional landscape can be just as complex and demanding. Emotional eating and stress are not just common topics heard in doctors' offices; they're part of many people's daily experiences. Understanding the triggers for emotional eating is key. Often, it's not hunger that drives us to the pantry but an emotional need. Whether stressed, anxious, sad, or even bored, food becomes a solace, a way to temporarily shield or distract ourselves from discomfort. For individuals like Tom, a retired banker and grandfather recently diagnosed with type 2 diabetes, stress from health issues and changes in lifestyle pushed him toward late-night snacks and comfort eating.

Tom discovered that his snacking was rarely about hunger. It was boredom and worry—worry about his health, and significant changes to his accustomed way of life. This realization was the first step in addressing his emotional eating.

The journey began with identifying patterns. His habit was to turn to sweet treats when reviewing his day, thinking about his dietary restrictions often triggered a rebellious, "Well, just one won't hurt" response. Recognizing this pattern laid the groundwork for change.

However, awareness alone isn't enough to break habits—especially ones that offer emotional relief. It requires developing new, healthier coping mechanisms.

Mindfulness practices played a central role in Tom's strategy. He started with mindful eating, a practice where he focused solely on his meal, savoring each bite and paying attention to the flavors, textures, and feelings. This helped him better recognize when he was truly hungry and when he was feeding his emotions.

Journaling was another tactic. By writing down what he felt when he reached for food, Tom began uncovering deeper emotional triggers and addressing them more constructively. Instead of eating, he'd take a walk, call a friend, or lose himself in his woodworking. These activities weren't just distractions; they were meaningful actions that helped him deal with emotions without turning to food.

Yoga and meditation also became vital tools. The breathing exercises helped him manage stress, a prominent trigger for his eating sprees. Over time, Tom found that by lowering his stress levels, his episodes of emotional eating became less frequent.

Support groups were a part of the solution, too. Sharing experiences and strategies with others facing similar struggles provided Tom the reassurance that he wasn't alone. This community aspect was crucial in maintaining motivation and gaining insights into managing his eating habits around his diabetes.

Of course, establishing a balanced diet conducive to diabetes management was fundamental. More frequent, smaller meals throughout the day helped keep Tom's blood sugar levels stable and reduced his cravings. Making sure each meal was satisfying both in taste and nutrition lessened feelings of deprivation that could lead to emotional eating. It's important to acknowledge that slips happen. Emotional eating is a behavior deeply ingrained in human psychology as a comfort mechanism. Tom learned not to be harsh on himself if he gave in to temptation but to view it as a learning opportunity. What was the trigger? How could he handle it differently next time?

Through a combination of mindfulness, journaling, physical activity, and support networks, managing stress and curbing emotional eating became integral parts of Tom's diabetes care plan. They were as critical as any meal plan or medication regimen because they addressed the root causes of behaviors that could derail his management efforts.

This blend of self-awareness, lifestyle adjustment, and community support can offer anyone a robust framework for managing diet and health. It's not merely the food on your plate but the thoughts in your mind and the emotions in your heart that shape your path towards wellness. Integrating practices to manage stress and emotional eating doesn't just help manage blood sugar levels—it enhances quality of life, turning the daily management of a chronic condition into a more holistic journey of self-care and health.

COMMUNITY AND SUPPORT NETWORKS

Navigating life with diabetes or prediabetes is akin to embarking on a challenging journey—one where the path is smoother and the load lighter with companions by your side. The role of community and support networks in managing diabetes goes beyond the occasional comfort; it is foundational to successful and sustainable lifestyle changes.

Imagine the story of Evelyn, a 58-year-old school teacher diagnosed with type 2 diabetes. The initial shock and overwhelm of her diagnosis were tempered by her proactive decision to attend a local diabetes support group recommended by her healthcare provider. This group met weekly, and through it, Evelyn found not just a wealth of practical advice but a sense of shared experiences and mutual understanding that she struggled to find elsewhere.

Support networks for individuals managing diabetes can take many forms, each serving unique functions. There are formal support groups facilitated by healthcare professionals, peer-led groups, online communities, and even less formal gatherings like cooking clubs or activity groups for those with similar health goals.

Informal vs. Formal Support Networks

Informal networks often include family, friends, and coworkers. They are the first line of emotional support—individuals who can offer a listening ear or a motivating word at a moment's notice. However, while invaluable, they might not always understand the nuances of the challenges faced by those with diabetes.

Formal support networks, on the other hand, fill this gap by providing structured support, education, and motivation in management strategies that are specific to diabetes care. They can offer a level of empathy and understanding that is deeply rooted in shared experiences. Typically, these groups also offer resources that might not be readily available in patients' immediate circles, such as access to specialists or information on the latest treatments and techniques for managing diabetes.

The Role of Technology in Support Networks

In today's digital age, online forums and social media groups also play a crucial role. They allow for a continuous connection with others managing similar health issues. For instance, Evelyn found an online community where members shared meal plans, celebrated milestones like reduced HbA1c levels, and offered advice on handling the side effects of medication. The 24/7 availability of such communities means support is available anytime, often right at one's fingertips.

Educational Workshops and Seminars

Beyond emotional and peer support, education is a critical element offered by these networks. Workshops and seminars can arm members with up-to-date knowledge about their condition. Whether it's learning about the impact of glycemic index on blood sugar levels, or understanding how to read food labels effectively, these educational sessions turn abstract concepts into practical, everyday skills.

The Psychological Benefit of Belonging

The psychological uplift that comes from belonging to a community cannot be overstated. It combats the isolation that many feel when first diagnosed with diabetes. Regular interactions with others who are facing similar struggles can provide a sense of normalcy and solidarity. For Evelyn, seeing others successfully managing their diabetes provided her with hope and a concrete belief that she could do the same.

Enhanced Motivation through Group Activities

Additionally, some support groups offer group activities like cooking classes or group exercise sessions, which not only teach valuable skills but also enhance motivation. Participating in a group walk or a shared meal preparation session can make sticking to a health regimen more enjoyable and less of a chore.

Navigating Challenges Together

Every journey has its setbacks, and the journey of managing diabetes is no exception. There are days when despite one's best efforts, blood sugar levels might spike, or a dietary slip-up occurs. In such times, the community provides reassurance and practical tips on how to get back on track without judgment or despair.

Evelyn's journey through managing her diabetes was significantly eased by her involvement in her support group. From learning about nutritional management to getting tips on incorporating exercise into her routine, each piece of advice was a stepping stone in her path towards health.

A Call to Leverage Community Resources

For anyone navigating the complexities of managing diabetes, tapping into these community resources can be a game-changer. Whether it's joining a local support group, participating in online forums, or simply starting a diabetes management club in your area, the value of these networks is immense.

By investing time in building and maintaining these support systems, individuals with diabetes can achieve not just better health outcomes but also enjoy a higher quality of life. The companionship, the shared knowledge, and the mutual encouragement found in these communities foster not just survival, but thriving in the face of diabetes.

CELEBRATING MILESTONES AND SUCCESSES

Embracing the journey of managing diabetes or prediabetes involves not just frequent blood sugar checks and nutritional adjustments, but also celebrating each step forward, no matter how small. The celebration of milestones and successes serves as a crucial element in sustaining motivation and fostering a positive outlook.

Consider the journey of Martin, a dedicated husband and father in his early sixties dealing with type 2 diabetes. Early in his diagnosis, Martin felt overwhelmed by the changes he needed to implement in his lifestyle. As time passed, supported by his healthcare team and family, he started setting small, manageable goals. Each time he met a goal, whether it was walking an extra thousand steps a day or skipping sugar in his coffee for a week, he took the time to acknowledge and celebrate these victories.

The Importance of Recognizing Achievements

Recognizing achievements, big or small, acts as a powerful reinforcement of positive behavior changes. It transforms the often daunting task of managing a chronic condition into a series of victories. This acknowledgment can be as simple as taking a moment to reflect on the progress made or as elaborate as organizing a small celebration. The key is to make these milestones noticeable and memorable, reinforcing the positive steps taken.

Setting Realistic and Personal Goals

Goal setting is inherently personal and should reflect one's lifestyle, capabilities, and eventual objectives. For Martin, it began with simple goals like choosing water over soda or planning at least one low-carb meal per day. As these became habitual, his goals grew more ambitious, such as maintaining his HbA1c below a certain level.

The Role of Support Systems in Celebrating Successes

The celebration becomes even more impactful when shared with a support system—family, friends, or even a digital community. Sharing success not only increases the sense of accomplishment but also encourages others in the community. When Martin shared his milestone of losing 10 pounds through better dietary choices, it wasn't just a personal victory; it inspired his peers, creating a ripple effect of motivation.

Integrating Celebration into Regular Check-Ins

Integrating celebration into regular health check-ins, such as doctor visits or diabetes education classes, can also provide professional acknowledgment of the hard work done. When healthcare providers highlight improvements in health metrics or adherence to treatment plans, it gives a technical validation to the efforts, adding a layer of professional satisfaction to personal victories.

Using Technology to Track and Celebrate Milestones

In today's digital age, various health apps and trackers can aid in both setting goals and celebrating achievements. These tools often include features that allow users to set reminders for medicine, track food intake, monitor exercise, and even link with others for shared goals and celebrations. When Martin marked six months of logged daily walks, his app not only congratulated him but also showed him a graph of his increased activity over time.

Addressing Setbacks Positively

Of course, the journey isn't without its setbacks. The manner in which setbacks are handled can significantly impact overall motivation. Turning setbacks into learning opportunities rather than reasons for criticism allows for continued growth and positivity. For instance, if Martin faced a week where he didn't meet his step goal due to a family commitment, instead of dwelling on the break in his routine, he reviewed what could be adjusted and set a plan to get back on track.

Establishing New Traditions

Celebrating milestones can also lead to the establishment of new traditions. For families, this might mean a monthly 'healthy recipe night' or an annual participation in a community walk for diabetes awareness. These traditions not only underscore the importance of sustained health management but also integrate fun and communal participation into what can be a challenging lifestyle adjustment.

The Broad Impact of a Positive Outlook

Ultimately, the act of celebrating milestones in diabetes management does more than just reinforce good habits. It fosters a positive outlook on life's potential, despite the challenges of managing a chronic condition. For Martin, each celebration was a reminder that his condition did not define his life's capabilities or its quality.

Inspiring Others Through Shared Experience

Celebrations shared in community settings have the added benefit of inspiring others. When people hear of someone achieving their goals, it provides tangible proof that the challenges they face can be managed successfully. It builds a narrative of achievable success that can encourage others to persist with their personal health goals.

Embracing these celebrations, sharing achievements, and setting new milestones— these actions form a crucial component of diabetes management. They transform a rigorous health regimen into a rewarding lifestyle, filled with recognitions and accomplishments that provide continuous motivation and joy on the journey to wellness. Celebrating each success is, in itself, a vital part of the treatment: a remedy that nurtures not just the body but also the spirit.

CLOSING REFLECTIONS: EMBRACING A NEW CHAPTER

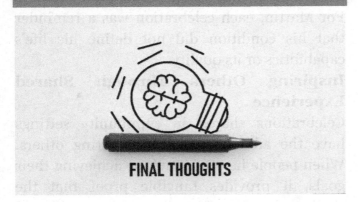

FINAL THOUGHTS

As we draw close to the end of our journey together in the *No-Fuss Diabetic Cookbook for Beginners*, it's essential to pause and reflect on the paths we've traversed and the new trails we're about to embark upon. Embracing a new chapter in life, especially post-50, often comes with its set of anxieties and uncertainties, yet it holds a boundless scope for revitalization and discovery, particularly when it comes to managing diabetes with a wholesome approach to eating.

Every beginning starts with an ending, and as you close this book, you're not merely finishing a series of chapters filled with recipes and guidance. You're actually opening the door to a new way of life—a life where health meets taste, and every meal brings you one step closer to wellness. We started by understanding diabetes and learning to craft meals that support your health goals. On this final page, let's envision where these newfound skills and knowledge will take you.

I began writing this book with one primary vision: to empower you to manage diabetes or prediabetes joyfully and deliciously. By now, my aim is that you've discovered not just a collection of meals but new habits and ideas that can guide you through this decade and beyond. Life after 50 can indeed be vibrant and fulfilling, and a substantial part of that vitality comes from the food you choose to eat, and the community you choose to share it with.

Imagine your kitchen as a new hub of activity in this fresh chapter of your life. It represents not just a place to prepare food, but a space where health is cultivated, where every ingredient you choose serves a purpose for your well-being. From the quiet stirrings of the morning as you prepare a balanced breakfast to the heartwarming smells of a family dinner, your kitchen is where the magic of transformation happens—an alchemy where raw ingredients turn into nourishment for both body and soul.

This transformation goes beyond your plates and palates. It extends to the very heart of how you view health and happiness. Managing diabetes isn't just about monitoring blood sugar levels or avoiding certain foods. It's about rediscovering the joy in meals that nourish and fulfill, creating a sense of abundance rather than restriction. Remember, a diagnosis doesn't define you; rather, it can refine you, guiding you towards choices that enhance your life in every aspect.

You've learned about balancing macronutrients, the importance of low-glycemic ingredients, and meals that can be enjoyed by the whole family. These principles don't just ease diabetic symptoms—they boost energy, help maintain a healthy weight, and enhance overall wellness. As an engaging part of your routine, cooking has hopefully become a cherished ritual that brings joy and health in equal measure.

I encourage you to keep the kitchen lights burning bright with experimentation and laughter. The recipes we've explored are more than formulas; they are stepping stones to innovation. Swap ingredients, try spices from different cultures, or maybe create a hybrid of two favorite dishes. Each successful experiment, each meal enjoyed by friends and family, is a celebration of your proactive stance towards a healthier life.

And remember, you're not walking this path alone. The community around you—whether it's family, friends, or fellow readers of this book—can be a tremendous source of support and inspiration. Share your new favorite recipes, perhaps start a cooking club, or host a potluck where healthy, diabetic-friendly meals are the stars of the show. As you share your story and your dishes, you might just inspire someone else to begin their journey towards health.

As you move forward, treat setbacks as learning opportunities. Not every day will be perfect, and not every meal will be a masterpiece. Yet, each challenge gives room for growth and fortitude, strengthening your resolve and deepening your understanding of your body's needs. Keep a journal of your culinary experiments and how they make you feel. This reflective practice can boost your motivation and help tweak your diet to better suit your evolving needs.

Above all, celebrate every victory, no matter its size. Each day that you choose health is a commitment to your longevity and well-being. Celebrate the quiet mornings spent crafting a nutritious breakfast, the gatherings around vibrant, vegetable-rich lunches, and the peaceful evenings that end with a sweet, guilt-free dessert. In closing, stepping into this new chapter with an arsenal of knowledge and recipes, remember the ultimate goal is not just to manage diabetes—it's to enjoy a full, health-oriented life that makes room for new tastes, new experiences, and new joys. Keep your spirit of adventure alive as you explore all the flavors and moments that await in this fresh, promising chapter of your adventure. Here's to good health, great taste, and a vibrant life. Cheers!

Made in the USA
Monee, IL
11 November 2024